Symptoms in Eye Examination

Symptoms in Eye Examination

Geoffrey V. Ball, RD, MSc, FBCO

Professor Emeritus, The University of Aston in Birmingham, England; Formerly Head of Department and Professor of Ophthalmic Optics, The University of Aston in Birmingham

Butterworth Scientific

London Boston Singapore Sydney Wellington Durban Toronto

First published 1982

© **Butterworths & Co (Publishers) Ltd 1982**

British Library Cataloguing in Publication Data

Ball, Geoffrey V.
  Symptoms in eye examination.
  1. Eye—Diseases and defects—Diagnosis
  I. Title
  617.7′154   RE75
  ISBN 0-407-00205-7

Typeset by Tunbridge Wells Typesetting Services Ltd
Printed and bound by Page Bros (Norwich) Ltd

Preface

In a time of increasing availability of automatic techniques in eye examination and in the use of computer-assisted methods for the analysis of data, it may not seem fashionable to write a book devoted largely to subjective manifestations arising from vision anomalies and other eye-related conditions, yet it is because of the emphasis on such developments that maintaining a balanced approach to patients and patient management has become necessary. Each day the practitioner is confronted by a sample of patients in the consulting room office or clinic; each exhibits the individual traits of personality; most have problems which must be probed through discussion, investigated by objective and subjective means and from the results of which decisions have to be made and communicated. Objective data, computer print-outs and pen recordings may help identify the cause of those problems and suggest how to relieve them, but the application of tests in variety must not override the simple observation that patients who attend for eye examinations are individuals, presenting their own problems in their own way, using their own idioms and hoping to leave reassured, with the cause identified and, where necessary, measures for relief of their problems put into operation.

If patients were prevented from communicating information then any examination resolves into the collection of basic data from which to speculate on possible symptoms. The symptoms predicted from that objective data might not be those which worried the patient most, nor might they have been identified at all. Communication with the patient, then, is the point from which all else commences; from which a sequence of operations develops based on sound scientific method designed to lead to the resolution of the difficulties which caused the patient to present for eye examination. If the patient has no problems but attends at predetermined intervals, discussion is just as important, for portents for their future visual welfare may become manifest.

This book is not immediately concerned, therefore, with physical measurements, nor with facts to be established only with the aid of computer visual display units or information retrieval services, interesting as they are in their own context. Neither is it a collection of symptom complexes nor syndromes. Ample literature is available on those topics. It is a book which is concerned with the interface between practitioner and patient in eye examination and with the seemingly simple, yet difficult art of extracting information by astute questioning, then sifting that information for relevance to the decision-making task. It is concerned with the patient as a presenter of individual eye and eye-related problems; with interaction between practitioner and patient, and with the importance of these influences in identifying and helping to relieve patient problems.

If there is one lesson I should choose to emphasize from all those learnt from experience it is to develop *active listening* — difficult to sustain patient after patient, week after week, year after year, but therein lies one major clue to competence in the evaluation of symptoms. Clinical competence comes from active listening to the patient, from personal experience, observation and reading, grossed up with the experience of others working in similar fields. The single-handed practitioner is at a disadvantage in that the opportunity for shared experience is lacking. This book may help in some way to make up for that lack.

Many texts advise that the patient should be questioned on mode of onset, intensity, duration and relationships of their symptoms, yet rarely give advice of the types of question and how they should be used in the history and symptom interview. I have attempted to correct that omission, for I should like this book to portray real life and not just the world of the lecture theatre. In places I have quoted examples of symptoms as they are described by the patient rather than transcribe those descriptions into the impersonal and cold language of the vision science laboratory.

Books, like statute law, suffer the constant danger of being out of date before the printer's ink has dried, and nowhere does this apply with more force than in the literature of science, medicine and technology. I decided early in my writings, therefore, not to attempt comprehensive reference guides. The scholar seeking references looks today more to computer searches, uses abstracting journals or the periodicals themselves rather than turn to references at the end of a book chapter. The general reader more likely looks for suggestions for further reading. Today there is a wide spread of journals relevant to vision and these are available quickly only to those with ready access to University-type libraries. I have indicated and acknowledged sources where this seems necessary or desirable and have given some recommendations for reading.

Some sections of the book are very closely concerned with eye examination and prescribing such as that on non-tolerance to optical prescriptions. Others are more generally applicable and are relevant to any health care practitioner involved in extracting and recording information from patients and then using that information for decision making.

Writing any book can be an absorbing task, but uninhibited writing like garrulous conversation contains repetitive and other superfluous material. Some drudgery and routine is therefore inescapable. Clichés have to be identified, deleted or rephrased; clumsy or over-long descriptions must be simplified; ambiguities removed. Nevertheless, apparent perfection in writing is fleeting. A deadline arrives when each sentence, paragraph and section has to be deemed complete, yet moments later some phrase or nuance of expression seems inexcusably naive or mistaken. I cannot expect to avoid these pitfalls or to be exempt from justifiable criticism by individuals in the various professions to which the book is directed. I can only request tolerance for any obvious lapses in the hope that these will not detract from the overall purpose.

Geoffrey V. Ball

Acknowledgements

Much of the material for this book has been condensed from lectures and clinical tutorials given during more than thirty years of undergraduate and postgraduate teaching. This teaching has been in association with colleagues from many different disciplines — general medicine, ophthalmology, psychology, physiology, physics, pharmacology, ophthalmic optics and optometry.

No book can be written in isolation from previous influences. Long forgotten discussions and conversations; ideas gleaned from general reading and literature searches; observations made by patients, clinical associates and students — all may be reflected in my writing and I acknowledge these influences even if I do not knowingly recollect them.

Clinicians, academics and researchers rely not only on their own studies and experience but also on the shared experience of others working in the same field and on other professions and disciplines. It is from the interplay of ideas in discussion that thoughts and views evolve and I offer my sincere appreciation for the stimulating discussions held over so many years to all my colleagues at the University of Aston in Birmingham, England. I am also indebted to the University for allowing me some months of study leave during which some topics were drafted. Especially valuable was the help received from Professor Graham Harding, Professor of Clinical Neurophysiology, who so ably took over the responsibilities of my University Department during my absence on study leave.

It was Reginald Lucking who in 1948 first persuaded me to become involved in teaching and who therefore is partly responsible for this book. Dr James Wilson encouraged and supported me in those early days and Dr John Austin shared the burden of clinical teaching with me for many years. Sadly, all are now deceased. Between 1954 and 1972 I gained very valuable clinical experience from long association in eye examination with Dr Robert Bolton, at that time Medical Officer to the University of Birmingham and from whom I learned much about the influence of psychoneurotic states in precipitating eye-related symptoms.

Professor Malcolm Gavin and, later, Professor Stanley Hunt both contributed to the development of ophthalmic optics and to the evolution of my University Department. The past advice of many others has been invaluable, particularly that of Professor W.D. Wright for his readiness to share so vast an experience ranging from colour vision to photometry at scotopic levels and Professor A.J. MacDonald (now regrettably deceased) for his help on the adverse effects of drugs.

Mr A.G. Sabell kindly took the photographs for *Figure 10.1* and the Graphics Design Section of the University of Aston were responsible for some other illustrations.

Many authors share responsibility for their views with eminent authorities who have agreed to comment on or modify parts of, or the whole, work and where experience and opinion are concerned the text tends towards the mean or accepted view. On the topics covered in this book the writings must stand on their own. The views, opinions and experience offered are mine alone and I would rather take, than shift, the full responsibility for the material which I present in the following pages.

Geoffrey V. Ball

Note on terminology

Various opinions exist on the interpretation and use of the words *optometry* and *ophthalmic optics* but I have used these synonymously throughout. Some may prefer one term or the other, but as I hope this work will have an international appeal I have, in places, taken *optometry* or *optometric* to avoid repetition and misunderstanding to a wide audience.

Notes on the tables

Summary tables in the various sections indicate some possible causes of particular symptoms likely to be met in a random catchment urban optometric practice in Great Britain. The tables are not intended to be exhaustive but to be used as a guide only in the hope that they may stimulate the reader into identifying additions or, maybe, deletions based on individual experience. These tables are then assembled in alphabetical arrangement as a reference guide in an Appendix.

Where conditions are considered to be of reasonably high incidence or the most likely reason for that symptom in the type of practice referred to above, they are placed high in a table. Exactly where a condition or group of conditions should be placed is, of course, debatable, but the incidence of some conditions is reasonably well established. Males with minor colour vision defects are common (6–8 per cent); females uncommon (0.5 per cent). The incidence of others would be generally acceptable from experience; for example, age-related lenticular changes; distance blur in corrected myopes needing a change in prescription; Mittendorf's lenticular spot — all would be classed as fairly high in frequency by any practitioner operating that kind of general practice. Others would be very low in incidence — nutritional-type amblyopia; acute glaucoma; clinically significant cyclophoria. Nevertheless, firm and diagnostically substantiated statistical evidence on the incidence of various conditions in optometric (ophthalmic optical) practice in Great Britain is lean and should be subject to further studies which would necessitate a comprehensive feedback of diagnostic information.

Contents

Part 1

The patient-practitioner interface in eye examination

Chapter 1

Introduction

The general nature of patients' eye-related problems and symptoms

Symptoms are generally considered to have either an organic or a functional base, that is, where a correlating change in body structure can be detected, the symptom is classed as organic; where not, as functional. The placement of a symptom into one of these two conventional categories is observer subjective and time dependent.

The detection of correlating structural change to account for a patient's symptoms depends on the experience, skill and methods of examination available at the time to the examiner. Disorders of function may signal a later organic change, or that organic change may be so slight on examination that no available technique can reveal it at that moment of time.

Most patients who attend for eye examination present vision or eye-related problems. These problems are usually, but not always, symptoms*. Some patients have no problems but attend at previously advised intervals. Others feel that re-examination is desirable having regard to the length of time since their last examination. Still others, and, as yet small in number outside health care screening programmes, come of their own volition for a first time precautionary examination.

Problems and symptoms

Some problems are symptoms, others are not. 'Am I likely to lose my sight because my mother did when she was sixty?' This appears to be a simple query rather than a symptom, but it discloses a state of mild anxiety.

'I have broken my glasses' is not a symptom *per se* but it is certainly a problem for that patient. The symptoms remain unstated until probed by the examiner. Sometimes problems arise only through the comments of others. 'When I am tired my friends tell me that I go cross-eyed, although I don't notice anything myself.' This constitutes an objective symptom or a sign (*see* Glossary on page 6), a perceptible change in the body or its functioning discernible to others but not to the patient.

---

*The decription 'problem' is interchangeable with the often used word 'complaint'. Complaint can mean a bodily ailment but it also has the connotation of a grievance. All health care practitioners see patients from time to time who feel that they have a grievance. In the context of eye examination this aspect is dealt with in Chapter 5 under the heading Non-tolerance to Optical Prescriptions.

Patients' problems, worries, observations and questions intermix with their symptoms and it is the task of the examiner to probe, sort and record logically and in abstract the major and minor difficulties from which the patient appears to be suffering. This is one function of the symptom and history interview.

A symptom is a subjective indication of disorder. Its expression is dependent on the integrated dynamic qualities which make up the personality of the individual patient. Symptoms must be communicated through words and idioms which patients find most appropriate to represent their feelings to the practitioner. Symptoms may not be present at the time of examination. Headache is a common symptom yet rarely is the patient suffering headache discomfort on examination. There is then the added difficulty for the patient of recalling these past inner experiences under the questioning of the examiner.

Words and expressions used by patients to describe their symptoms may seem to them to be relevant and succinct but they may not be to the examiner. All experienced practitioners will have been astonished at times by the peculiar descriptions and strange analogies arising in the course of a history and symptom interview, and some of these are considered later. The more elaborate and dramatic the phrases used in recounting symptoms the more are they suggestive of a neurotic temperament.

Concepts in symptom reporting

Consider the common report by a patient 'I get headaches'. Is the 'ache' to this patient likely to be the same as to another? Almost certainly not. It will differ in potency, quality, duration, location and so on. But, is the *concept* of an ache to the patient the same as that to the examiner or, indeed, to any other patient? Again, in some measure almost certainly not. Furthermore, is the examiner's concept likely to be exactly that of another examiner? Once more, this is doubtful. Nevertheless, although there will be individual differences and nuances of interpretation this shared concept has a common verbal definition for a certain type of feeling. Patients expect the practitioner to understand that peculiar type of feeling and also expect that intelligible information has been communicated in so describing their symptom in that way.

This philosophical treatment emphasizes that different sensations arising in different patients may be reported in the same terms; equally that the same sensation may be reported differently by different patients, or possibly even by the same patient at different times.

Some terms commonly used by patients in eye symptom reporting include: ache, pain*, blur, dizzy, weak, tired, strained, clear, and so on. In questioning the patient it is therefore important for the examiner to encourage patients to elaborate on the concepts and terms used in describing their problems as indicators to reliability, powers of observation and introspection, vocabulary and personality.

The ability to investigate and to make valid deductions from all the problems, including symptoms, as described by patients is one characteristic expected of the competent physician, optometrist, ophthalmic optician and ophthalmologist. As routine skills become automated so will more time become available for the less tangible skills of communication from which are derived the subjective problem-

*There is sometimes discussion as to whether words such as 'ache' and 'pain' should be referred to as 'sensation', that is, as elementary experiences, or as 'perception'. Perceive and perception are now used most frequently in the context of 'becoming aware of external objects' rather than in the older, more general sense of 'becoming aware of' so that the word 'sensation' is more appropriate.

specific data for each patient. Once determined, the objective and subjective data will be capable of rapid analysis by computer-assisted techniques to predict significance. This will allow greater certainty in diagnosis and referral, thus benefiting the patient, the optometrist, the general medical practitioner and the ophthalmologist alike.

Primary and secondary symptoms

It is often possible to identify a primary or main symptom (chief complaint) from the history and symptom interview. Where a primary symptom can be distinguished then other symptoms are classed as secondary or subsidiary. The main symptom is that which is of most concern to the patient and which usually has led the patient to seek advice. However, the main symptom may not be the symptom having the highest weight in clinical decision making. For example, a patient's chief worry may be difficulty in close work such as is normally experienced by those over the age of 45 years. The symptoms having the greatest significance to the examiner may be the occasional blurring of vision with vague eye discomfort. The main symptom therefore need not dictate the final action but it cannot be ignored. If no proposal is communicated to the patient to deal with their primary symptom then dissatisfaction may result and any optical prescription, however carefully determined, may be rejected psychologically.

It is also very useful to refer to the main symptom in any letter or report where a patient is being referred for attention by other health specialists.

Symptoms of obscure origin

The aetiological probabilities must always be borne in mind whenever there is no immediately apparent explanation for a patient's symptoms, that is, where the aetiology is obscure then high incidence anomalies should be eliminated as a possible cause of symptoms before considering those of low incidence.

Discomfort in or around the eyes is more likely to be due to minor psychological stresses than to the interesting, but rare, syndromes dealt with in a teaching curriculum. The recent onset of impaired vision as daylight fades might be caused by early primary pigmentary retinal dystrophy, but in general practice the highest probability is that of a mere myope needing a change in prescription. In patient care, therefore, where the cause of symptoms is not manifest, a routine should be followed in problem solving which considers the relatively high probabilities first, examining for and eliminating each in turn.

'Simple' before 'complex' should be the rule in such cases and this applies just as much to the methods of examination to be used in the later investigations. How far consideration of some of the low incidence conditions will proceed will be limited by individual specialization, knowledge and experience and by the rules which guide practice at the time in the particular country or state.

Through fear of complaint or fear of legal action, through anxiety brought about by unbalanced emphasis in teaching, practitioners can become ultra-cautious, and so unreasonably, that extensive regimens of complex investigations are instituted based on minimal guiding information. With the exception of well organized and controlled health care screening, there must be good reason to suspect disease before subjecting the patient to elaborate, time-consuming and often uncomfortable investigations.

Glossary

Symptom   Subjective evidence of disorder or disease (subjective symptom*).
Sign   Objective evidence of disorder or disease (objective symptom*).
Symptomatology   The science of symptoms.
Symptom complex   The collective symptoms of a particular disorder or disease.
Syndrome   The collective symptoms and signs characteristic of a disorder or disease.
Organic symptom   A symptom with correlating manifest anatomical lesion.
Functional symptom   A symptom without observable correlating anatomical lesion.
Presenting symptom   A symptom which the patient presents (to the practitioner).
Main (primary) symptom (chief or major complaint)   The symptom which gives the patient greatest concern.
Subsidiary (secondary) symptom (minor complaint)   Any symptom other than the main symptom.
Guiding symptom   A symptom which leads to a diagnosis.
Latent symptom   A sign which precedes a correlating symptom.
Referred (sympathetic) symptom   A symptom manifested in a part of the body other than that from which it originates.
Problem   A difficulty (presented by a patient.)
Complaint   (1) A bodily ailment or symptom reported by a patient. (2) A grievance presented by a patient.

---

*The modern usage of 'symptom' is restricted to subjective observations only, that is, those of the patient. Earlier, both objective (signs) and subjective (symptoms) observations of disease were intended in the expression 'symptoms of disease', hence the term 'objective symptom'. Most non-medical dictionaries define the word in this all-embracing but historical mode. Sometimes 'objective symptom' is used in the sense of a sign from which the presence of a symptom may be deduced.

Chapter 2

The art and science of the history and symptom interview

Clinical history and symptom investigation is part art, part science. The art is in extracting the relevant information from the patient and guiding the patient along the routes which seem to be most productive. The science is in recording, interpreting and analysing the data so that the subsequent examination can be best directed to establishing a provisional diagnosis. The history and symptom interview is not only an occasion for collecting data about vision and the eyes although that is one main aim. This discussion has a wider purpose. The patient interacts with the examiner, but this represents no more than the interplay of personalities from which it is simple to make intuitive judgements which may not be justified. There is no time in a normal eye examination to apply lengthy scientific methods to study the behaviour of the patient. However, it is essential to establish as good a rapport with each patient as is possible in the limited time. The good clinician must be part actor, part counsellor, part therapist, part educator, part philosopher, part psychologist, part social worker and a first class refractionist.

The garrulous patient has to be restrained by well-timed intervention; the shy patient must be coaxed to provide information; the aggressive patient must be calmed with polite firmness and the anxious patient set at ease with kindly reassurance.

The introverted optometrist must occasionally act out the sociability of extroversion and the extrovert optometrist must sometimes taste the apprehensions of introversion.

Of all the health professions those concerned with eye examinations are able to devote more time than most to communicating with the patient and this is an opportunity to educate and to counsel as well as to analyse, diagnose and to treat.

The interview has a therapeutic value. 'A worry shared is a worry halved', so the saying goes. It is rare for a patient to have the opportunity to talk to someone who is willing to listen, comment and advise on their visual and other troubles. This acts as a valve for the relief of tension. The importance of becoming an active listener; the importance of concentrating on the patient as the symptoms and concerns pour out and the importance of making succinct and relevant comments are demonstrated. Sometimes the patient is parodied as saying 'it is so nice to go to see him. He's very, very attentive and I always go there . . . I can't get on with his glasses though . . .' So, the practitioner, whilst mindful of the therapeutic value, must not neglect the other important clinical aspects of professional work, otherwise the parody may become reality.

Apart from the gathering of data, the history and symptom interview has other functions, some of which are as follows.

(1) It allows the examiner to observe the patient and to make judgements on such characteristics as personality, motivation, attitude, speech, mannerisms and physique and gives some indication of the reliability of the patient's observations.

(2) It develops the examiner's powers of communication, interpretation and deduction.

(3) It indicates general, optical, ophthalmological or other medical abnormality which may suggest special emphasis and conserve time in the later examination.

(4) It gives initial pointers to the relative urgency of action.

The patient as a research project

Each new patient can be thought of as a research project in miniature. Problems have to be stated; hypotheses have to be studied, tested and discarded; data has to be collected; significance has to be considered and provisional decisions made and confirmed. The various stages to be completed for each patient, not always in the same order include the following.

Collection of data.
Identification of problems from the data.
Collection of additional problem-oriented data.
Analysis of data.
Provisional decisions/diagnoses.
Confirmation of provisional decisions and diagnoses.
Proposals for action and/or treatment.
Confirmation of action and/or treatment.
Continuing care and advice.

The immediate task is to collect information from the symptom/history discussion so that the patient's problems can be identified.

Methods of data collection in the history and symptom interview

The data may be collected in one of several ways.

(1) Verbally and directly from the patient, notes of which are then entered on to record cards or sheets: on to problem-oriented records or the data is processed for later access by microcomputer.

(2) Questionnaires completed by the patient before or during interview.

(3) Taped conversations with the patient.

(4) Video-sound recordings.

Conventionally and conveniently the data is usually collected by questioning the patient directly and by entering on a record card or sheet. (3) and (4) are rarely used in the consulting room office at present although the taping of conversation (with the patient's permission) may assume greater significance in the future. Storage of and access to information in a readily accessible form will become easier with the computer-assisted record systems. Formal details such as full names, addresses and occupations are sometimes obtained by other personnel in the practice, such as a receptionist. If this is done the importance of *accuracy* in recording such details must be stressed in their training.

Types of questions used in the history and symptom interview

Several basic forms of question must be used during discussions with patients, defined as follows.

Open-ended question

A question which provides a simple frame of reference, yet gives maximum freedom for expression and reply.

Funnel questions

A series of questions which commence broadly but successively narrow to specific points.

Problem-oriented question

A question designed to probe a particular problem or symptom.

Closed question (fixed alternative question)

A question to which the patient has the choice of certain well-defined answers only.

Leading question

A question which, by its wording, is suggestive of the reply.

Direct question

A question in which the matter on which information is sought is posed in the wording.

Indirect question

A question in which the matter on which information is sought is *not* posed in the wording but which is designed to lead to disclosure of the desired information in the reply.

The use of types of question in clinical interviews and examinations

Open-ended questions are most frequently used in the early parts of clinical interviews. They are designed to allow patients freedom to talk about their problems in their own words. Later, more specific questions must be asked; fixed alternative, indirect, and so on, so that the basic and problem-specific data can be collected if this has not been possible from the initial open-ended questions. An open-ended question is sometimes better than a direct one.

An examiner may note, for example, that the patient is wearing some kind of bifocal and wishes to check whether any difficulties have been experienced with bifocal prescriptions. The obvious and simple direct question is: 'Do you have any difficulty with your bifocals?' A better frame of reference is provided by an open-ended question such as: 'I see that you are wearing bifocals. Some people find them excellent; others have some difficulty with them . How do you feel about them?' The patient should not now feel abnormal or exceptional if having to admit to problems and is more likely to disclose and discuss these problems. The practitioner can then funnel the questions into more precise areas of bifocal wear depending on the answer to that open-ended question. If the patient admits to problems when negotiating steps, for example, then the examiner may use direct questions such as:

'Do the steps look blurred?' (Yes, no, sometimes, undecided.)

'Do you notice the dividing line between the distance and near part?' (Yes, no, sometimes, undecided.)

Closed and leading questions are also useful during clinical examinations but the latter must be used with caution. The crossed cylinder technique has closed questions to which there are three possible answers — (first position; second position or neither). The crossed cylinder technique also involves leading questions. The examiner may initially indicate two choices only — view one and view two. After several applications to which the patient has given a distinct choice, that choice will become less emphatic as visual equality approaches. At some point a leading question such as . . . 'or are they about the same' must be injected. However, it is better to give this third alternative in the original statement of information to the patient or to remind the patient of the fixed alternatives as the examination proceeds.

Indirect questions are important in note-taking as one way of avoiding suggestion in susceptible patients. Care must be taken in mentioning special symptoms such as halos around lights and photopsia for some patients will agree to the suggestion through confusion, hypochondria or other neurosis, through uncritical acceptance of the idea or just because they wish to be congenial. The over-cautious practitioner could be driven by anxiety or stress into elaborate and complex investigations. If it is felt that direction needs to be given to the patient who might otherwise have difficulty in remembering visual problems other than their main worries then it is wise to interject an indirect question or to leave the specific question until later in the examination when rapport will have developed with the patient. This is particularly important where the patient has given no grounds for suspicion and the symptom is specific to a low incidence condition (*see* Chapter 10).

The psychology and semantics of patient management

How the examiner communicates with each patient is just as important as the methods of examination used and the successive steps by which a provisional diagnosis is reached (Chapter 3). After the preliminary data sheet (face sheet) details of name, forenames, etc., have been completed the first clinical question directed to the patient is of crucial importance both in its phrasing and in the manner of its presentation. Most patients have problems and want to tell the practitioner about them in their own way and in their own time. If the interview is conducted along rather formal directive lines, that is, the questioning is more or less fixed, then the patient becomes frustrated as the examiner asks questions which seem irrelevant to their main worries.

Commencing the interview

Except in special situations, some of which will be mentioned, the open-ended question is the best introduction for the history and symptom interview. In a hospital or clinic the initial question may have to be different. The history and symptom recording is often carried out elsewhere in such institutions so that case notes are already available. Nevertheless, the case notes recorded by one practitioner will not be identical to those of another although there should be agreement on the main symptom, if one exists. Case notes covering ophthalmological aspects may not have established all the optical details so these may have to be expanded.

Information on many aspects of vision and the eyes must be obtained from all patients and it is most agreeable to the patient to begin the interview with a very general open-ended question. This serves a dual purpose: it allows the patients to unburden their worries immediately and gives the practitioner an opportunity to observe reactions, demeanour, habits, attitude, choice of words, and so on. This open-ended question can take many forms. It should be simple and easily understood, not too formal but such as to retain that necessary element of control of the interview.

Suggested questions are indicated in the verbal schedule at the end of this Chapter. Most patients are concerned with a few simple issues such as: (1) to relate their eye and vision problems; (2) to ask the cause of their problem(s); (3) to find out what can be done; and (4) to know whether what can be done will be painful, either physically or financially.

The desirability of commencing the interview with a general and non-specific question may seem obvious but it has been known for students to ask as their first question: 'Have you ever been to an eye hospital or had eye operations?' And it is informative to find the reasons for such a question being given priority at the beginning of an optometric examination. The concensus seems to be that the possibility of eye disease is so important that it should override all else. The possibility of eye disease *is* important and the patient must be questioned on that and on any previous hospital treatment at some time during the discussion, but only at a stage where the practitioner has had time to establish rapport. The psychological impact must be considered in patient management. The average patient attending in general practice will not have thought of eye operations, nor of hospital, and may be worried by the possible reason for that question posed starkly at the beginning of the interview. The patient may feel that some obvious and possibly serious eye condition is so apparent to the examiner that an immediate question on eye disease has been precipitated. The question is inappropriate at the opening stage in general optometric practice and should be left until later in the discussion.

The responsibility for the detection of eye and related disease can be overstressed by clinical instructors so that students develop a fixation on this aspect at the expense of all others. The patients' interests are best served by a realization of the need for such questions, of the relative incidence of eye disease, but also of the need to establish good communication with each patient and to avoid anxiety-producing situations.

Stereotyped phrases and questions must be avoided. Similar questions have to be put to all patients in the collection of basic data but it is useful to make subtle changes in their presentation from patient to patient. If this is not done then questions become automatic and the patient who is wearing glasses is nonplussed when they hear the practitioner ask: 'Do you wear glasses?' It is essential that the examiner looks directly at the patient when delivering the opening question, but this may sometimes be forgotten in the hurly-burly of a busy practice or by students in training. Following the answer to this first question the patient can be funnelled along different problem-oriented routes by supplementary questions designed to obtain data not previously covered by the patient's answer to the opening question. If the practitioner uses a check list of basic information requirements then the various points can be checked or ticked as they are covered (*Table 2.1*).

For the initial part of the interview a schedule of basic questions is needed which is best written down, but which usually exists only in the examiner's mind. Although most examiners would not choose to read out these questions verbatim there is a

TABLE 2.1. History and Symptom Interview — Abbreviated Aide-mémoire

Vision: dist., near., cent., periph., binoc., monoc., phot., scot.
Other visual symptoms.
Eyes: adnexa.
Discomfort: pain.
Referred: headaches.
Eye diseases/treatment.
Optical : medical : family histories.
Medications.
Occupation : visual tasks : recreations.

danger of accidental omissions becoming permanent. A written schedule ticked off for each patient is one method of avoiding omissions, or if that is unacceptable to the individual practitioner a written schedule should be kept for regular reference. Problem-oriented questions will vary depending on the problem and therefore no single simple set supplementaries will be suitable for every patient, although supplementary question schedules which are problem-oriented can be built up for each problem or symptom by the individual examiner.

It is most common to find no check list for the history and symptom interview on printed record cards, although there are often simple check lists for objective examination; for example, media, fundus, pupils. The only check point relating to history and symptoms on many cards is 'date of last examination'. An abbreviated aide-mémoire is given in *Table 2.1.*

The extension of history and symptom note-taking throughout the examination

The history and symptom interview does not end when the basic and problem-specific information has been discussed and written down, at the beginning of the eye examination. Patients may make diagnostically significant comments at any time during the examination. The examiner must therefore not be afraid to repeat questions to which the answers have previously been equivocal, but if such is the case it is best to change the wording so that the patient is not immediately conscious of the repetition. This has the added advantage of checking patients' responses.

Patients do not recollect all their eye and vision experiences at the time of the original questions. For example, the examiner may find a small corneal nebula during focal illumination which could have resulted from the removal of an embedded foreign body at some time in the patient's history. An appropriate question will already have been asked during the history interview (for example, 'Have you ever had cause to go to your doctor about your eyes or to a hospital?' To which the answer was 'no').

At this later stage, on noticing the corneal nebula the examiner would interject:

'Do you remember ever having anything in your eye like a piece of grit or metal which had to be removed?' It is hoped that this will trigger the patient's memory. It often does.

Typical schedule designed to satisfy the basic data requirements of the history and symptom interview

General open-ended question relating to eyes and vision

The answer to this general open-ended question may cover some of the following data but the information should be obtained for all patients.

Present state of central vision (patient's opinion)

(1) Distance: binocular, monocular, photopic, scotopic. (Specific: blur, loss, unease.)
(2) Near: binocular, monocular, in artificial lighting.

Present state of peripheral vision (patient's opinion)

(1) Photopic. (2) Scotopic.

Other visual symptoms

Open-ended question. (Specific: diplopia, photopsia, halos, floaters, colour vision, metamorphopsia, chromatopsia, photophobia.)

Eyes and adnexa (patient's opinion)

Open-ended question on symptoms associated with eyes. (Specific: (1) discomfort: for example, 'hot' or 'cold' eyes, dry, watering, discharging, gritty, itchy: (2) pain.)

Asthenopia

Referred (sympathetic) symptoms

Specific: headaches, drowsiness, vertigo, dizziness, nausea, confusion.

Eye diseases and/or treatment

Conditions, operations, injuries, forms of treatment.

Optical history and symptoms

(1) Adequacy of present prescriptions (patient's opinion). (2) Last eye examination: date and by whom. (3) Last prescription (glasses or contact lenses): date and by whom. (4) Glasses or contact lenses worn constantly, intermittently, distance only, near only. (5) Occupational use. (6) Other optical treatment (for example, L.V.A. devices, C.C.T.V. etc).

General medical history

Open-ended question on general health. (Specific: illnesses; hypertension; allergies; trauma.)

Present medications

Specific: tranquillizers, antibiotics.

Family history

Open-ended question on family eye problems. (Specific: for example, glaucoma, strabismus, myopia, diabetes.)

Occupation and recreations

Working conditions, lighting, hazards.

Verbal question schedule designed to satisfy the basic data requirements of the initial history and symptom discussion (colloquial language — suitable for many patients)

(1) (*a*) Are you satisfied with your vision or your glasses at present?
      (*b*) Do you have any special reasons for having your eyes examined?
      (*c*) How do you feel about your eyes, your glasses or your vision at present?
Such general open-ended questions do not introduce the concept of *difficulties* or *problems* at that stage but give the patient a simple *neutral* frame of reference — eyes, glasses (*a*) and (*c*), or neither of these (*b*).

(2) (*a*) Are you satisfied with your distance vision out of doors in the daytime (with your glasses)? And, outside at night? And, how do you find your vision with each eye?

   (*b*) What is your vision like for reading and close work (with your glasses)? And, indoors at night?

(3) And your side vision? Out of the corner of your eye?

(4) Have you noticed anything else about your vision at all? (Specific examples may be injected here if the practitioner feels this necessary: for example — halos, flashing lights, visual distortion, etc.)

By now some degree of rapport will be established with the patient and questions can become more specific.

(5) Do you have any other trouble with your eyes? (If problems have been reported earlier.) (Specific examples may be used: for example — watering, discharge.)

(6) Do your eyes seem to get tired?

(7) Do you get headaches? (If yes — specific problem-oriented questions on headaches: *see* Chapter 8).

(8) Have you ever had anything wrong with your eyes needing treatment by your medical doctor or in hospital?

(9) How are you getting on with your present (distance) (reading) (bifocal) glasses (or contact lenses)?

(10) How do you keep generally — your general health?

(11) Do you take any medicines or tablets regularly?

(12) Have any of your family or immediate relatives ever had any problems with their eyes? And your parents or grandparents? Do you know if they had any eye trouble? (Specific examples may be injected with caution.)

Notes

When the answers are obtained to the main questions they may have to be further elaborated by additional problem-oriented questions derived from the special sections devoted to those problems.

At a few points in the initial interview it is useful to interpose the patient's name in a mode suited to the particular practitioner, practice, office, country or state.

It is convenient and useful for both practitioner and patient for a concise verbal summary to be made by the examiner at the end of the formal history and symptom interview along the following lines.

'So, the main reason for having your eyes examined seems to be that you have problems in reading . . . having to hold things further away to see clearly and very occasionally dull headaches above your eyes?'

Further reading

BANNON, R.E. (1952). 'Symptoms and case history . . . the patient as a person.' *Am. J. Optom.,* **29,** 275–285

BERNSTEIN, L. and DANA, R.H. (1970). *Interviewing and the Health Professions.* New York: Appleton-Century-Crofts

Chapter 3

Communication with the patient

The hallmark of a competent scientist is, if called upon, to be able to explain his work to any person varying from academic colleagues to his neighbour's children in language which those individuals are likely to understand. Respect gained apparently by obscure terminology, mystery and aloofness is, in the end, no respect at all and is the trademark of the charlatan.

A good exercise in the power of communication is to attempt an explanation to a lay person of some commonly used technical term such as heterophoria or the fraction 6/6 (20/20). At the simplest level, this fraction could be explained as representing normal vision for a certain age, but that is somewhat evasive. The real test is to explain both the numerator and denominator separately, and it is the latter which gives the greatest problem for a patient who has no knowledge of subtenses, visual angles and so on. A possible explanation is appended as a footnote*.

Where some disagreeable procedure or condition has to be communicated then the thoughtful practitioner must consider carefully the choice of words to be used in the discussion with the patient so that the possibility of stress being generated, apparent discourtesy or offence is minimized. It is a matter of considering probabilities rather than there being any ultimate certainty that this, or that word or expression will or will not be acceptable to the patient.

Words and phrases which seem to have a high probability of causing distress or offence must be identified and avoided.

For example, older patients, certainly in Great Britain, are still liable to link a word such as 'deficiency' with the old concept of 'mental' deficiency and no patient will

---

Numerator The distance to the chart of letters in feet or metres (the use of a mirror in reversed methods may have to be explained).
Denominator Simply, the distance at which letters of a (demonstrated) size are just read by a person with average vision. If there needs to be a more detailed discussion then (pointing to a 6/60 ((20/200)) letter), 'This very large letter can be read easily at a close distance by a person with average vision, but if it is taken far off into the distance there comes a time when it can only just be made out. If that distance is 200 feet or 60 metres then that size of letter is given the number 200 or 60. A very much smaller letter might just be made out at 20 feet or 6 metres and that letter would be given the number 20 or 6. So the lower number is the furthest distance at which a person with average vision should just be able to read a letter of that size.' (Average vision might simply be described as being determined from many investigations of vision on many different people.)
The whole 6/6 therefore means that at 6 metres distance (the top number) the person has a standard of vision which allows them just to make out letters which are also just recognized by the person with average vision at that same distance of 6 metres written as the lower number.

relish being referred to as 'defective' or 'deficient'. Also, the older patient is not likely to react favourably to the word 'senile' which, once more, has a connotation of loss of mental faculties. Traditions can change, of course, and optometrists must be alert to the changing customs and language in their particular country or district.

Abnormal, subnormal, deficient, defective, all have an element of stigma when applied personally, yet these are commonly used to describe various conditions. Other examples are suggested in *Table 3.1*.

TABLE 3.1. Some Emotive and Phobic Words Best Avoided in Discussion with Patients, Unless the Patient Uses the Description First

Abnormal(ity)	Defective	Hysteria
Anno domini	Deficiency	Paralysis
Atrophy	Degeneration	Senile
Blindness	Growth (as in des-	Stronger (as of myopic lenses)
Cancer	cribing tumours)	'T.B.'
Cataract	Haemorrhage	Tumour

'Senile macular degeneration' is a particularly bad term to use within the hearing of patients because of its two emotive words, as also is 'senile cataract'.

These descriptions become even more distressing if they are overheard by patients to whom they do not apply but who assume that the reference is to themselves.

Note Words such as 'cataract' and 'haemorrhage' fall into a special category. With health education they should lose some of their present phobic quality. If these words are avoided by practitioners it can be argued that this will perpetuate the present position. It will sometimes be necessary therefore to make use of a word such as cataract but always it is best to precede its use by an explanation of the true nature of the condition. For example, in a patient who has no special knowledge at all: 'Inside your eye is a lens which is usually quite clear and transparent. In your (left) eye this lens is becoming less clear so that some of the light is being cut off and your vision now isn't quite so sharp in that eye.'

Variation, difference, modification, are better words for the patient/practitioner interface.

Examples

Avoid
Your vision is subnormal (6/9).

You are colour defective and confuse some colours.

Some suggested alternatives
Your vision doesn't quite reach average levels.

You have a somewhat modified form of colour vision. Certain distinct colours tend to look much the same to you.

Technical jargon

Technical phrases or words will not convey the same meaning to lay patients. Some words or phrases are so commonly used in ophthalmic science or ophthalmology that they occur unnoticed in the practitioners conversation and lead to confusion and possible anxiety in the patient unless the ground has been prepared by a preceding simple explanation (*see Table 3.2*).

TABLE 3.2. Some Common Technical Words Used in an Ophthalmic Context Which are Best Avoided in Discussions with Patients Unless or Until they have Special Knowledge

Aberration	Case	Foreign body	Prognosis
Accommodation	Confrontation	Fundus	Reflex
Acuity	Cylinder	History	Refraction
Addition	Deficiency	Media	Refractive error
Axis	Field	Monocular	Sphere
Base	Fix	Objective	Subjective
Bichromatic	Fixation	Orbit	Tension
Binocular	Fogging	Prism	Test types

Common words and phrases likely to confuse the patient

Some patients, either because they are less alert due to age or through nervousness, take time to interpret common phrases or words which are well understood under normal circumstances. 'Left' and 'right' are confused through orientation problems in a darkened consulting room. The astute practitioner quickly decides whether to use those designations or different but more expressive descriptions such as (in the examination for heterophoria): 'Is the line towards me or towards the door?' The intelligent patient who, because of nervousness, confuses elementary responses, is spared the embarrassment of admitting to apparent stupidity. Some common adjectives are best discarded because their interpretation differs widely and involves judgement of value.

'Have you ever had any serious eye problems?' To the practitioner, 'serious' may seem explicit. Information is being sought on conditions such as retinopathies, glaucoma, strabismus, eye operations and not on simple errors of refraction. The patient may interpret 'serious' in this way but more likely the fact of having to wear glasses is a 'serious' problem. If the patient answers 'yes' to this question it has to be probed further and in many cases will bring forth only the history of refractive error. 'Serious' is a relative term — relative to the involvement of the person in eye-related matters.

Accuracy in questions or descriptions to patients

It is very easy to lapse into imprecision in describing techniques to patients largely through continual involvement in the methods of examination. For example: 'Look at the red and green circles' when directing attention to a bichromatic Landolt Ring test. In truth they are broken black circles on red and green backgrounds. Some patients understand the practitioner's verbal shorthand; others are sensitive to such inaccuracies and, not wishing to make mistakes, ask 'Do you mean the black circles with gaps on red and green?' The examiner, corrected, seems rather foolish. One other example is illustrated by the question: 'Can you make out the bottom line of letters?' when the practitioner means 'Read the bottom line of letters.' The truthful patient whose vision does not permit them to identify the letters replies 'Yes, I can make them out', following which the examiner has to give the proper direction 'Now will you read them to me'.

The word 'refraction' is not used synonymously with eye examination outside optometry, ophthalmology and medicine; indeed, physicists and scientists generally interpret the word as a simple optical phenomenon. 'I am going to look at a refraction' may mean something to an optometrist but to one trained in elementary physics it could be interpreted as pushing a stick into water and watching its apparent bending.

Avoiding lengthy or ambiguous questions, repetitive words and phrases

The long question in nearly always a bad one. The maxim should be to reduce questions to as few words as possible. It is a good exercise to tape an interview (with the patient's permission) then transcribe the questions on to paper. The questioner can then delete, change or alter the order of words at will. By re-recording these new question models the interviewer, alone or with colleagues, can decide which are best suited to which type of patient. The only justification for long questions is where sufficient information must be provided so that the patient can understand and be in a position to reply to that question.

Ambiguity in questioning — the overuse of common words or expressions — is not always appreciated by the questioner until the interview is recorded and played back. The number of 'wells', 'you knows' and similar clichés may surprise. This may irritate the patient but ambiguity in questioning is confusing and more serious. 'Is it better or worse in position one or two?' asked during an examination with the crossed cylinder method, needs supra-alertness on the part of the patient if equally confusing replies are not to be elicited.

Use of the patient's name

Addressing the patient by name during the examination is fundamental to establishing rapport but is easily forgotten. The daily appointments list should be checked before each patient enters the consulting room and the optometrist should always know the name of the next patient. Greeting the patient by name is the first step to good patient management. The patient's name should then be used occasionally but not too frequently during the examination.

Avoiding the stop-go interview

Interviews with patients should flow naturally and not be subject to continual hesitations whilst the examiner enters details in the case record or thinks of the next question. Early in a student's training in case history investigation it is common to observe difficulties being experienced in asking questions and writing down information from the answers. The interview becomes question — answer — silence (whilst information is entered in the record), and this cycle is repeated very many times.

Good interviewers cultivate the ability to look back and forth at the patient, listen to information, abstract the essential detail mentally and write this down in brief whilst posing the next question. Sometimes the information given by a patient in answer to a question may be lengthy yet so important that the examiner feels this must be written down in full and without interruption. If so, it is best to keep the patient informed of the reason for a long silence by interjecting a comment such as 'I'll write that down before I go on'.

The patient who has not had a previous eye examination

Most people have an eye examination at some time in their lives. On the first occasion they are likely to be mildy apprehensive although most will not outwardly show this. The patient does not know the examiner and knows little or nothing about the methods used in the examination, particularly whether these methods are uncomfortable or even painful. Their nervousness may be enhanced by the psychological impact of a consulting room which has the air of a dental surgery.

Patients who have had a previous eye examination are likely to remember a little about the kind of observations required and the methods used. The first-time patient must be treated with especial care. It is more than ever necessary to give an explanation or reassurance before each new method of examination. This applies with force to such techniques as ophthalmoscopy where the examiner has to approach very close to the patient or where bright lights are to be used.

'Wrong' and 'right' answers

Patients become concerned about whether they have given a 'wrong' answer in subjective testing. 'I hope I am giving you the right answers' is a common plaintive comment and calls for reassurance. The patient must be advised that the decisions do not rely solely on their answers and that results are double or treble checked. They can be assured that objective methods (which can be simply explained) give a good indication of the information needed.

The 'bottom line of the test chart'

The design of test charts is a matter of personal preference but a good design allows for each line of small letters to be exposed singly so that patients do not become alarmed if supra-acuity letters for their age cannot be read.

6/7.5 or equivalent represents good vision for many patients over the age of 70 years but if the succeeding lines of 6/6 and 6/5 are exposed at the same time the patient becomes very conscious of not reading more than the 'third line up from the bottom'. There should not be a 'bottom line' of the test chart used in the consulting room. This is easily arranged where projection methods or drums are used.

Assertions made by patients

It is unwise to disillusion older patients by deliberately setting out to demolish their long-held beliefs even where these seem to be quite mistaken, yet the examiner should never agree with statements for which there is no evidence. It depends whether the patient makes an assertion or asks a question. What can be done is to side-step the issue without agreeing or disagreeing. For example, if the patient purely needs a reading addition for simple presbyopia: *Patient:* 'Of course, I have ruined my eyes by reading in bad light.' *Examiner:* 'So, you do quite a lot of reading then?' But, if the patient asks the question: 'Do you think I have ruined my eyes by reading in bad light?' Then the examiner should give the answer that there is no evidence for this occurring and that it is normal for a reading addition to be needed beyond a certain age.

In younger age-groups there is a somewhat greater case for challenging statements like those above, as a contribution to health education, but in the ageing patient, visual habits and beliefs acquired over a lifetime are not easily changed, and unless the practitioner has ample time available it is best to proceed with the examination rather than enter into discussion which is most likely to be unprofitable.

An intriguing and sometimes disturbing feature of clinical life for any practitioner occurs when a patient makes assertions with emphasis and often pride such as: 'I have a very unusual condition in my left eye.'

The experienced practitioner will try, by subtle questioning, to get additional clues, but this kind of patient is often delighted to keep the examiner guessing — playing a kind of clinical 'hide and seek', by withholding information. It is the greatest relief on examination of the eyes to find some fairly obvious, often congenital, condition for which there need be no concern. Persistent pupillary membrane, hyaloid remnants, papillary crescents are but a few. Frequently the patient has reported the wrong eye; frequently also, even after the most careful examination of both eyes everything appears normal. The patient may pursue the examiner with questions such as: 'Haven't you found it yet?' and the newly qualified are likely to become tense and ruffled. They need not do so. This type of patient may be best pleased, particularly with a young practitioner, to be able to explain this so-called 'unusual' condition, usually in garbled terms. 'The last person who examined my eyes told me that it would prevent me from going blind' is the kind of statement which might puzzle at first. However, it should soon be apparent that the patient refers to a cilio-retinal artery which a previous examiner must have pointed out. It is unwise to bring such normal appearances to a patient's attention unless there is some special reason for so doing, such as an explanation for the retention of central vision after some vascular catastrophe.

Communication with patients on methods of examination

It is always desirable to give patients a brief description, suited to their background, of any special method of examination to be used. Reassurance that the method will not prove painful, if this is the case, should be offered, particularly to young and elderly patients. Keratometry may be taken as an example.

If, from the symptom and history discussion, the patient has demonstrated alertness and interest, yet has no special or technical knowledge, then the preamble to keratometry could take the following form.

'This instrument is called a keratometer and it measures the curvature of the cornea, that's the clear, curved part of the front of your eye. It's perfectly comfortable for you and you won't have to answer any questions. I shall watch the reflections of these lights and take measurements and all you have to do is to look at the green light in the centre. Now, put your chin on this rest, head right up against the bar, and do you see the green light? Good, keep as still as you can, it will only take a few moments.'

It all sounds condescending when read out from this kind of written statement, but that is how an examination method should be introduced to a new patient. The patient has no idea at all of what is about to happen, whether it will be painful, and may be very nervous when confronted with some complex-looking piece of apparatus.

Etymology of technical terms

In the example given above, a patient who has some scientific background might ask why the instrument is called a keratometer. An examiner who never knew, or has forgotten the etymological principles of their special language appears particularly inept when confronted by that type of patient. In a random catchment practice, the next patient might be a professor of physics or a local housewife and each is capable of asking demanding questions. It is prudent to anticipate the unusual response. An etymological optometric or ophthalmological dictionary is one essential book for the examiner's library.

Health education

Practitioners involved in eye examination have more time with individual patients than in many other medically orientated professions. Often, an examination is relatively simple where, for example, a patient has been seen many times before and is attending for regular re-examination. Time is available for the communication of health education matters. Issues must not be pressed unduly but the opportunity exists for enlightening patients on vision and eye problems generally. Obvious examples include colour deficiency, refractive errors and other common eye problems. Any example chosen should relate directly to that patient or have a bearing on their visual future, such as presbyopia. Patients should be encouraged to ask questions about vision and eyes and to develop a healthy intelligent approach to these matters in the hope that established and incorrect dogma may be eradicated. There is, for instance, a common lay view that cataract is 'something which falls down behind the sight' reflecting not just the derivation of the term but also common medical opinion of two hundred years or so ago.

Myopic patients

All experienced ophthalmic practitioners will have examined spectacle wearers, usually myopes often from oriental origins, who have memorized the 'number' of their lenses using words such as angle for axis. 'The number of my lenses is . . .' and the main concern is whether the number has increased or not. Herein lies one of the important and psychologically significant aspects of myopic semantic therapy.

Glasses do not increase — they change. The number is different, a slight difference is needed now to give best vision and, assuming that it is, vision is perfectly normal with the new prescription. The low myope has lenses at the bottom end of the range in the trial case or refracting unit and the practitioner can show the patient that many myopes need lenses much further into that range.

Spectacle wearing myopes sometimes move their head rather than their eyes as a way of avoiding the unwanted optical edge effects of certain forms of lens. Uncorrected myopes may be described as having a 'detached' look probably resulting from habitual under-accommodation for near objects with its associated under-convergence and possible monocular central suspension in situations where the refractively normal individual accommodates and converges correctly. The resulting 'far off' appearance has been said to give certain myopic actors and actresses a peculiar attraction and enhanced popularity in films and television prior to the widespread use of contact lenses. Similarly, 'he is far away' is a regularly heard description for the facial expression of a normal person who has relaxed convergence rather than fixing the speaker.

Reactions of patients to some techniques of eye examination

Throughout any eye examination a patient may make comments about visual appearances or react in ways which are informative and significant to the final assessment and decision. Some reactions can seem to be quite peripheral to the task in hand at that time, yet they convey important indicators to the experienced examiner.

Indicators derived from patients' observations of letter charts

A line of letters may be read backwards by normal patients if the examiner is using a reversed method of examination (that is, a mirror at ten feet or three metres), but this could also indicate bitemporal hemianopia. Small areas of central field loss cause a patient to misread letters, for example, E may be called F, or they may miss out some letters on a line. Commencing or finishing reading in the middle of a line can also suggest central field loss. These problems may be disclosed by the patient in the history and symptom interview and should be noted as needing special attention later in visual field investigation.

A child having normal visual acuity reads compacted letters slowly but usually correctly, such as from the six metre line of a typical letter chart. Letters which are separately presented, as are available in some special tests, will be read quickly.

Letters are described as double when they are merely blurred and are said to 'come and go' in fluctuations of accommodation or in central field loss. Letters appear marginally smaller with low over-correction of negative power, and marginally larger with minor positive over-correction.

It is mildly unnerving, especially for the newly qualified when, after an uneventful objective examination such as retinoscopy, a patient can see but cannot read even the largest character of the test chart, and nothing in the prior investigations has suggested this.

The first advice to the examiner is to consider the simple explanations first — accidental misplacement of a cylindrical axis in changing to subjective methods, the patient is not looking in the correct direction, an incorrect lens has been inadvertently left in place. Apart from these obvious reasons, the problem occurs in fairly large hypermetropic errors when monocular subjective examination is attempted following retinoscopy (that is, fellow eye occluded). Accommodation is relaxed somewhat under the conditions of retinoscopy but is re-exerted immediately on monocular examination, demonstrating the need in this type of refractive error for some form of binocular examination. Alternatively, there may be long-standing amblyopia which has not been uncovered by the previous discussion or investigations, or poor vision for some other reason.

Coloured fringes to black characters are described by patients when in a state of blurred retinal imagery. The effect disappears when the retinal image is sharp.

Occasionally, when directing a patient to read their best line of a letter test chart where all the lines are exposed simultaneously, the patient reads no identifiable line to the confusion of the examiner who knows all lines from experience. The confusion could occur through the examiner's inattention; alternatively, the patient has begun by misreading several letters, has begun in the middle of a line or is reading backwards. It is wise not to communicate confusion to the patient by a direct comment so that confidence is sustained. It is better to inject a direction such as 'now read the line above that one' in order to give time for re-orientation.

Other reactions or comments

In measuring the near point of convergence, the patient who has convergence insufficiency frowns and attempts to retreat from the advancing test object whereas the normal patient smiles or laughs openly as the point of extreme convergence approaches.

In subjective examinations it is common for patients to apologise if they have to change an observation, probably from the established opinion that there has to be a right and wrong answer to every question of the examiner. For instance, in a muscle balance test where the patient must identify the position of an arrow or line the response goes: '. . . on number two — no — sorry, it's on four — sorry, no — it's moving.' Reassure the patient that it is quite normal for movement to take place but that the line or arrow will probably settle at a fixed place.

If some eye deviation takes place under cover during the cover test, then, on uncovering the occluded eye the patient often blinks as an aid to re-alignment of the visual axes. This interferes with the close observation of eye movements and the test must be repeated following instructions to the patient not to blink.

Retinoscopy in a semi-darkened room is an excellent soporific, particularly in older patients, and should be completed rapidly if the patient is not to become quite sleepy. This is a common fault with students and the newly qualified, whereas experience suggests that rapid decisions in retinoscopy will give the best results.

Distraction during the examination

It is difficult for most practitioners to concentrate on parts of the eye examination which demand special care if a conversation has to be sustained with the patient about the methods being used as they are being carried out. A few patients are particularly inquisitive and demand to be told about retinoscopy, muscle balance techniques or bichromatic tests and interject questions into the examiner's own question routine. Command of the examination must be politely maintained otherwise faulty results are encouraged by distraction. Each examiner must develop individual gambits to restrain such patients so that attention and concentration can be given to the task in hand but it is important that all such gambits shall be truthful. An instruction repeated several times in succession followed by silence has the effect of quietening a garrulous patient for a time. 'Now look at my light . . . keep looking at my light . . . straight at the light.'

Alternatively, most patients would be unhappy if wrong results were the consequence of interruptions of the examiner's attention so the point can be made with some force because it is quite truthful. 'I'm sorry, but I can't talk at the moment because it might cause me to get wrong results.'

For similar reasons it is difficult to examine close friends or relatives who insist on commenting on the examination, on the room decoration or on personal matters. It is a common occurrence for 'grief cases' to be found amongst optometrist's relatives or close friends and unintentional distraction during the examination is one likely cause.

It is worthwhile working out personal procedures to fit the individual style and personality of the examiner so that authority is maintained without causing offence.

Communication of clinical decisions

Some practitioners argue that firm decisions should always be given to patients on all major matters, because equivocation, they suggest, may lead to a loss of patient confidence or, worse still, be interpreted as incompetence.

In many types of patient firm decisions are possible. A patient in the mid-forties complaining of discomfort in near work together with an increased working distance and with no other symptoms or signs, demonstrates such classic evidence of the effects of normal loss of accommodation due to age, that a firm decision on the need for an optical prescription and of its potential for the relief of symptoms can be taken and communicated to the patient. Many other types of patient fall into similar categories, including the simple myope with the sole symptom of distance blur and all other functions within normal limits. The verbal certainty which can be given to these patients can, unwittingly, be extended to less certain cases.

Firm decisions are desirable at all times where there is reasonable supporting evidence or experience for that decision, otherwise a simple honest statement of the position should be given. There can be no long-term satisfaction, for example, in directing a patient to wear lenses with the verbal assurance that symptoms will disappear if that possibility is uncertain. The symptoms may well subside for a time as a placebo effect helped by the accompanying dogmatism, but if the optical or binocular vision problem is not the precipitating factor then they are likely to recur. Placebos have a place in optometric practice as in general medicine (*see* Chapter 5) but they must be used sparingly and not as an excuse for avoiding communicating difficult decisions in clinically difficult patients. The acquisition of unsubstantiated prescribing dogma must be guarded against especially by practitioners who work single handed due to the lack of opportunity for critical discussions of techniques and clinical decisions with others working in the prescribing field.

Reassuring the patient

It is often possible to detect anxiety in patients who have close relatives with eye problems or eye disease. If the patient reports such events, particularly early on in the examination then it is more than ever necessary to give reassurance if there proves to be no cause for concern. Some typical and common examples are as follows.

'Our family have always had poor eyesight.' 'My eyes have always been very weak.' Very likely these comments refer only to inherited simple-type myopia. Reassurance should be given if the patient has age-norm visual acuity, along the following lines. 'Yes but with the proper glasses your vision is perfect.'

'My father went blind with cataract when he was in his sixties.' Reassure of normality if there are no signs. This type of observation is frequently made when the patient is much younger, often in the thirties or forties.

'I have never been able to see very well with my left eye.' Sometimes this proves to be a fairly high refractive error with resulting long-standing amblyopia or sometimes a minor myopic/astigmatic error in the affected eye which reduces vision lower, but often not much lower, than 6/6 (20/20). In the case of monocular amblyopia, reassure the patient by stressing the normality of visual acuity with the other eye (if this proves to be the case). In conditions such as minor correctable refractive errors which give normal visual acuity emphasize that vision with the correct prescription is perfect.

Obsessional behaviour

Patients sometimes develop obsessional behaviour about their eyes and vision; for example, monocular visual acuity, the optical performance of glasses, or their fit. Obsession about the corrected vision of each eye is very common. In a variety of situations the patient can be seen covering off or shutting one eye after the other, comparing, contrasting, judging minutely the appearances and returning regularly for possible re-examination and advice.

A fixation can develop on the orientation of an astigmatic correction. The patient regularly examines the prescription, tilting this way and that to check whether some minimal shift would marginally improve vision — a shift of such minor degree that it can be nullified instantly by the manner in which the glasses are put on or by interference from the hair.

How does the eye practitioner deal with such patients? It can be argued that if no significant optical error or other abnormality are found then the patient is deemed neurotic and sent elsewhere with little or no discussion. Such actions discount the therapeutic value to such patients of attention and communication. A person willing to listen and comment on their symptoms and problems in private, acts as a relief valve for inner tensions. Within the limits of the time scale of eye examination, the optometrist and ophthalmic optician can perform a valuable health care service to the patient even if the decision to refer the patient back to their own medical adviser was made quite early in the examination.

There can be no routine or rules to govern the management for every patient, but the following are general observations on handling these situations.

(1) Retain composure, even if the patient's problems appear vexatious and trivial.

(2) Listen to the patient's comments. Do not dismiss them immediately. There may be a genuine problem obscured by a weight of irrelevancies.

(3) Do not censure the patient, even if the temptation is great.

(4) Give the patient truthful, yet simple, observations on their problems.

(5) If a solution is proposed give a simple explanation of the suggested course of action.

There is a possibility that a practitioner who gives time to such patients will reap a harvest of neurotic individuals gravitating to the practice. It is equally probable that the practitioner who dismisses all such problems as time-wasting will acquire a reputation for brusqueness, even of discourtesy. In the final count it is the personality of the practitioner which will determine the interaction, or lack of it, with such patients but it is a matter of judgement as in most things in life; the avoidance of extremes in behaviour and in contacts and communication with other human beings.

Very rarely it will be necessary to tell a patient firmly that they are wasting time but the practitioner must be sure that reasonable measures have been taken to investigate the problem and to send the patient for other advice where clinical investigation and judgement shows this to be desirable. Sometimes, however persistent the examiner in questioning the patient, no significant information can be gained other than the main complaint of vague discomfort (*see* Chapter 6, Visual Unease). If initial observation shows there to be no obvious injection, then the course of action can only be to follow the normal investigation pattern giving special attention to those parts of the examination which provide indicators for urgency in further investigation such as possible early retinal detachment. If all observations and data are within normal limits judged from the practitioner's experience there is no reasonable cause to suspect eye or related disease. Such patients may be wise to have a general health care examination and the eye practitioner must bear this in mind when giving final advice.

Further reading

GREGG, J.R. (1969). *How to Communicate in Optometric Practice.* Philadelphia: Chilton Book Co.
LEVINE, N.R. (1976). 'Improving student understanding and management of patients through role-playing and video-taping.' *Am. J. Optom. physiol. Optics,* **53**, 2, 95–99
WICK, R.E. (1970). 'Communication as an optometric technique.' *Am. J. Optom.,* **47**, 9, 720–728

Chapter 4

Recording of clinical data

Clinical data recording has arrived at a crossroad as this book is being written. Conventional and long-standing systems such as individual record cards which have served professions well for a century or more can now be replaced by sophisticated clinical data storage/retrieval systems with access by keyboard and information on visual display. These recent developments may revolutionize traditional clinical record keeping but it is too early yet to predict their eventual impact, particularly for the individual practitioner. Their use in clinical research and in assisting in medical diagnosis is already well established. Because of these innovations and their potential impact in the next few years, only a brief survey of clinical recording in optometry is given here.

Clinical data recording in optometry and ophthalmic optics still rests largely on the old-established, well-tried record card or sheet mostly handwritten, stored in conventional filing cabinets or drums and retrieved manually when required. For some time ahead the majority of single-handed practitioners will continue to use manual recording and retrieval if for no other reason than the cost of hardware and software if full use is to be made of micro-computer assistance to the practice. The economics of the introduction of computer assistance have to be judged, for example, against the merits of updated or new clinical equipment for eye examination where finance is restricted.

Clinical record systems

Clinicians differ in their preferences for examination techniques and nowhere more so than in the details of clinical data recording. A record system designed to satisfy the needs and preferences of one clinician is unlikely to satisfy entirely the needs and preferences of any other clinician. Individual choices also vary with experience so that whatever the basic method used there must be flexibility to allow for change, particularly for shifted emphasis or innovation in the examination routine. If a traditional printed record card is favoured then some space should be left unclassified so that information can later be inserted without costly reprinting.

Record systems designed for research, for the teaching clinic or hospital must be distinguished from those intended for the single-handed practitioner. The requirements of clinical data recording for research purposes are not covered here. It is always necessary to decide the protocol in advance. Optometrists considering using their clinical data for potential research studies must always seek advice on the research design unless that skill has already been acquired.

Photo-documentation as a method of monitoring the progress of conditions is important, particularly as a safeguard in possible litigation. Fundus and slit lamp photography are readily available, but expensive, techniques for the individual practitioner.

Main purposes and requirements of clinical records

In the early months of practice it is possible for the young practitioner to recall many details about individual patients without extraordinary feats of memory. As experience lengthens and with the day-to-day demands of practice, most of the elements of each eye examination are lost to recall as soon as the next day's appointments commence, or even before that, unless there were some extraordinary symptom, prescription, event or patient. All experienced examiners have a mental collection of notable eye examinations, patients or prescriptions stored for immediate recollection when required — unusual prismatic or astigmatic corrections, very high refractive errors, 'grief cases', bizarre patients — but few could recall individual details about those patients who need merely a common presbyopic reading addition or some minor myopic distance prescription.

One main purpose of a record system, therefore, and one which is rarely emphasized, is to help to recall the patient at some later stage, hence the desirability of writing down personal notes on each patient — personality, hobbies, recreations, habits and idiosyncracies — all in a code if necessary as a safeguard should the record be lost.

There are more obvious reasons for good record keeping. These include the following.

(1) Conforming to legal or ethical requirements. In Great Britain, under the National Health Service Acts the maintenance of adequate records is mandatory.

(2) Progressively recording changes in the state of refraction and/or binocular vision.

(3) Identifying significant changes from previous findings which might indicate the need for further investigations.

(4) Assisting the practitioner in developing and maintaining an acceptable routine of examination.

(5) Assisting the practitioner's defence in the event of litigation.

(6) Providing continuity of information on dispensing and other areas related to good practice management.

Record systems

Record systems can be grouped under three headings, as follows.

(1) Record cards or sheets, usually printed, allocating space for each part of general eye examination and related matters together with space or supplementary cards/sheets for additional examinations.

(2) Problem-oriented systems.

(3) Computer-assisted systems designed for recall by visual display or print-out.

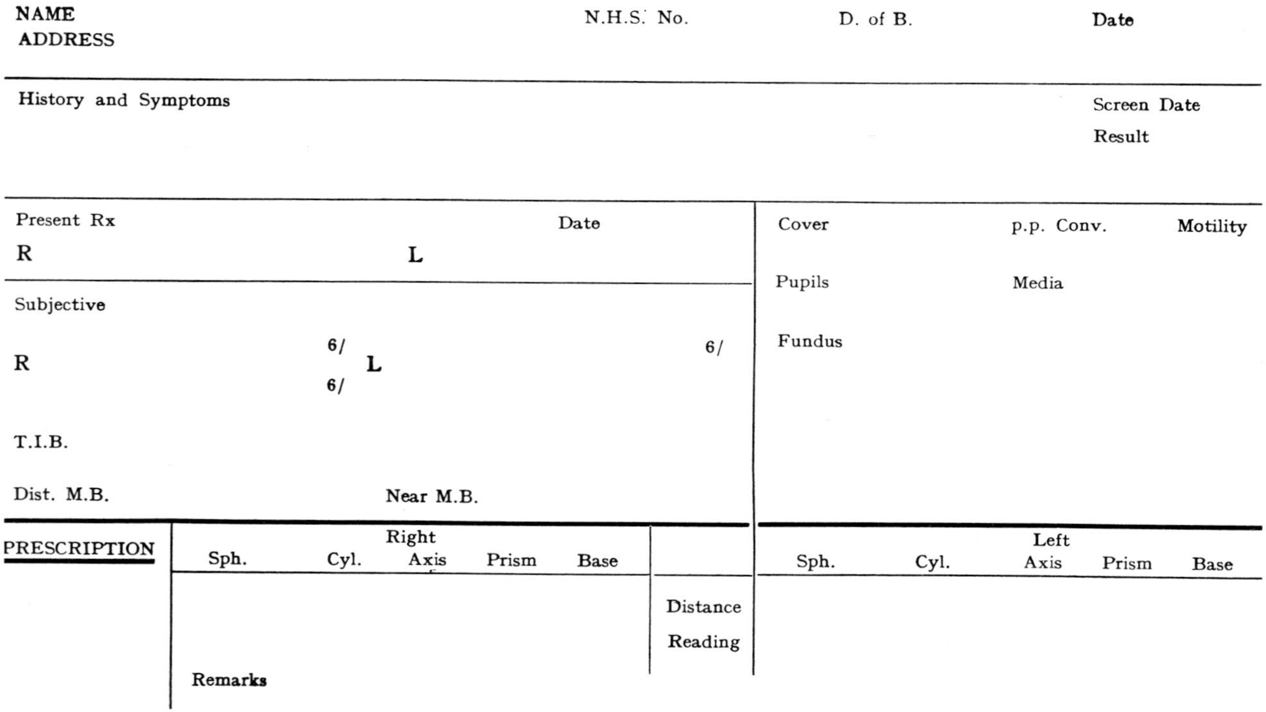

NAME
ADDRESS

N.H.S. No.

D. of B.

Date

History and Symptoms

Present Rx
R   L   Date

Subjective

Cover

Pupils

Fundus

R   6/   L   6/
         6/

T.I.B.

Dist. M.B.   Near M.B.

PRESCRIPTION		Right						Left		
	Sph.	Cyl.	Axis	Prism	Base		Sph.	Cyl.	Axis	Prism	Base
						Distance					
						Reading					

Remarks

p.p. Conv.   Motility

Media

Screen Date
Result

Figure 4.1. Record card designed by the author (c. 1957) for use in a health centre

Notes

(1) A predetermined requirement at that time was that the section 'prescription' should fit the dimensions of the same section of the British National Health Service prescription form (O.S.C.2) so that a carbon copy of the prescription, exactly as written, could be taken, for use should later problems arise in interpretation with the authorities.

(2) Dispensing was not carried out in the health centre.

Record cards

In designing any conventional clinical record card many variables have to be considered and the most important is the basic examination routine for which the record is intended. Once the data base has been laid down then the space to be allocated for each part of the examination has to be decided within the overall permitted dimensions of the card. This is so individual a matter that no one else should be responsible for the design than the practitioner who is to use the system. If a group of clinicians is involved in that use, then unanimity is unlikely. Either some compromise has to be worked out in discussion or the clinical leader must decide the detail having regard to the individual views. What is essential is that a pilot study be

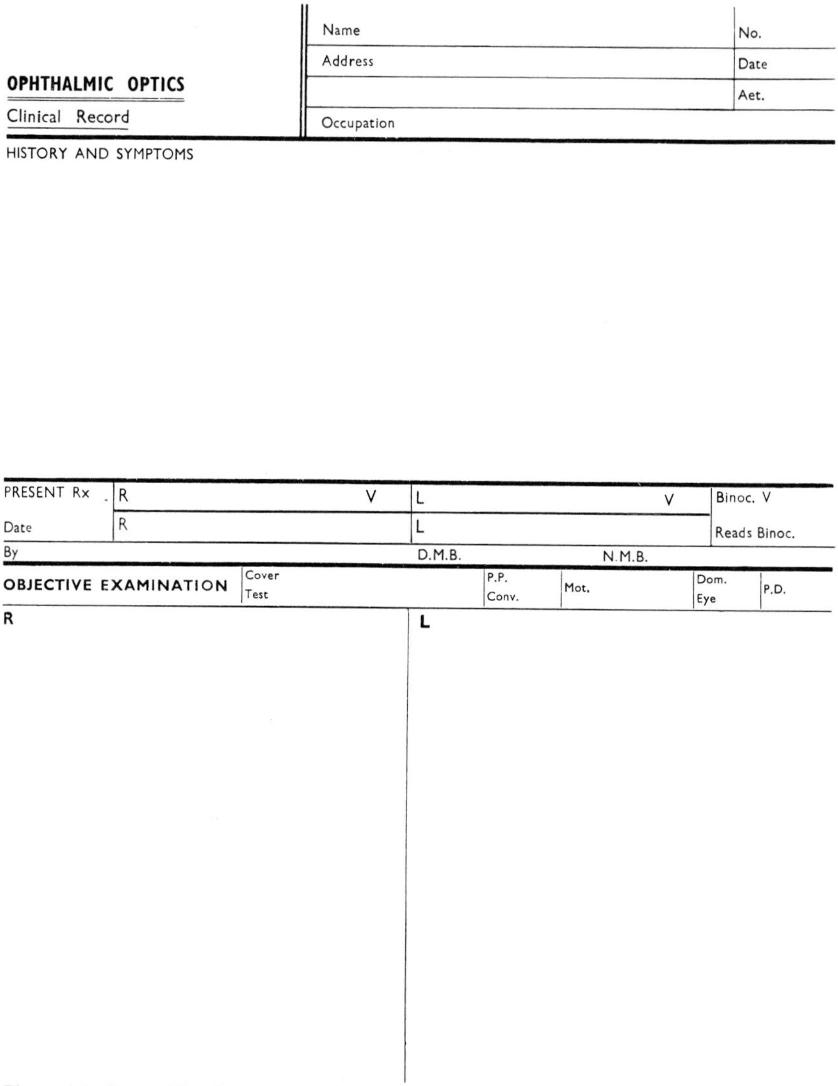

OPHTHALMIC OPTICS	Name	No.
	Address	Date
Clinical Record		Aet.
	Occupation	

HISTORY AND SYMPTOMS

PRESENT Rx .	R	V	L	V	Binoc. V
Date	R		L		Reads Binoc.
By			D.M.B.	N.M.B.	

OBJECTIVE EXAMINATION	Cover Test		P.P. Conv.	Mot.	Dom. Eye	P.D.
R			L			

Figure 4.2. Front side of a record card designed by the author (c. 1958) for use in an eye examination teaching clinic *(continued)*

carried out with any proposed new printed record so that problems in use can be identified and the layout changed before the costly exercise of final printing is embarked upon. It is also very desirable that a printer's proof should be obtained in advance otherwise words such as ophthalmoscopy or symptoms will most likely be misspelt.

One example of individual style is shown in *Figure 4.1*, and a record card designed for use in an eye examination teaching clinic is illustrated in *Figure 4.2*. Record cards for the eye examination/dispensing teaching clinic have to be extensive and elaborate and have to cater for many different types of examination usually as addenda to the main record. Filing space is usually not so limited as in the average practice, or the

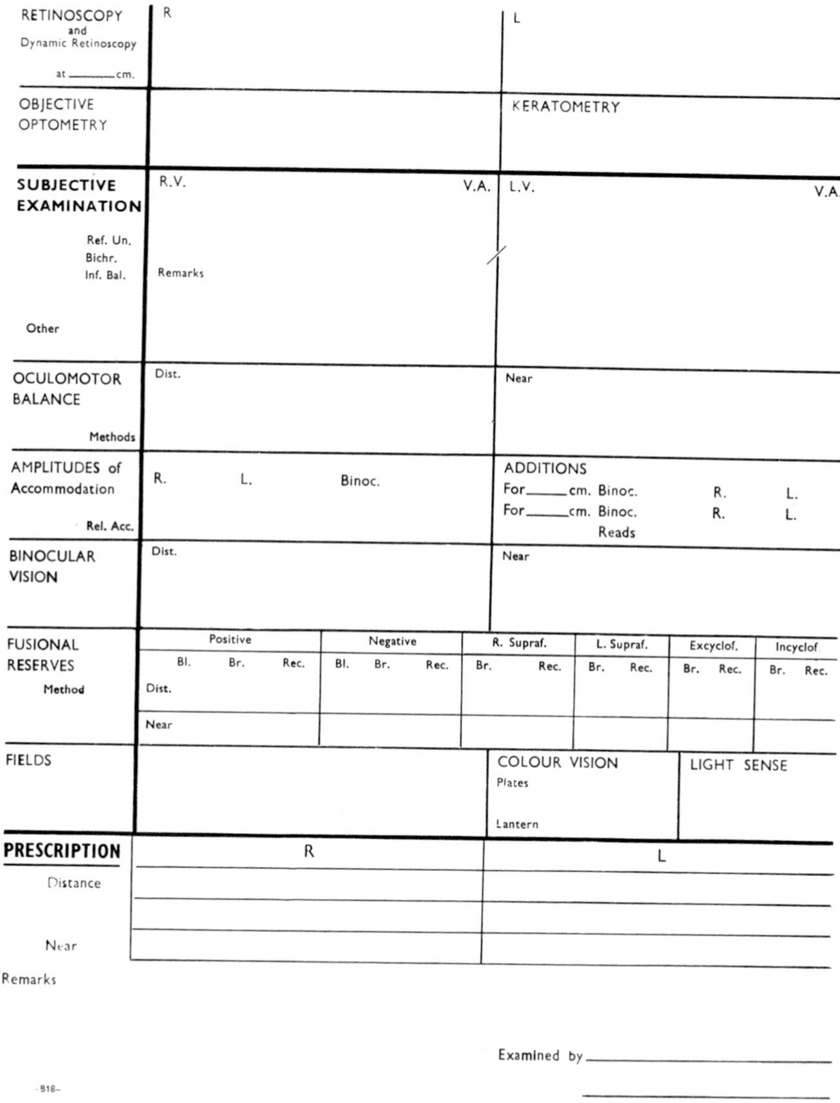

RETINOSCOPY and Dynamic Retinoscopy at ____cm.	R				L				
OBJECTIVE OPTOMETRY					KERATOMETRY				
SUBJECTIVE EXAMINATION Ref. Un. Bichr. Inf. Bal. Other	R.V. Remarks			V.A.	L.V.				V.A.
OCULOMOTOR BALANCE Methods	Dist.				Near				
AMPLITUDES of Accommodation Rel. Acc.	R.	L.	Binoc.		ADDITIONS For____cm. Binoc. For____cm. Binoc. Reads		R. R.	L. L.	
BINOCULAR VISION	Dist.				Near				

FUSIONAL RESERVES Method	Positive			Negative			R. Supraf.		L. Supraf.		Excyclof.		Incyclof.	
	Bl.	Br.	Rec.	Bl.	Br.	Rec.	Br.	Rec.	Br.	Rec.	Br.	Rec.	Br.	Rec.
	Dist.													
	Near													

FIELDS		COLOUR VISION Plates Lantern	LIGHT SENSE

PRESCRIPTION	R	L
Distance		
Near		

Remarks

Examined by _____

-B1B-

Figure 4.2 (continued). Reverse side of the record card shown on the facing page

older records can be transferred to microfilm. Some of the special features for which separate cards or sheets must be provided include: low vision aid analysis, binocular vision/orthoptic investigation, dispensing, aniseikonia investigations, colour vision examination (*see also* Problem-oriented systems).

The most telling criticism of record cards generally, such as that shown in *Figure 4.2*, is that they are technique-orientated or test-orientated and encourage a 'box-filling' mentality. Whilst useful in the early stages of a student's career as a means of having some order in teaching, too complex a 'boxed' record card has many disadvantages for both patient and practitioner. One of the perennially difficult problems for all those involved in eye examination is the decision on data to be collected for *every* patient. Recent views are tending towards keeping this to minimum levels with less emphasis on the *routine* examination, which has had so great an influence in the past. This is one reason for the shift towards considering more the problems of the patient rather than the problems of the examination routine.

Problem-oriented systems

Problem-oriented systems extend the more conventional methods of examination and recording in that they are designed to shift greater emphasis into identifying and monitoring patients' problems[1]. This emphasis derives from a data base from which a problem list is developed, leading to a plan of action and progress notes for each problem identified. The data base includes both 'defined data', that is, information obtained for every patient, and 'problem-specific' data or information relevant to the problems identified for the individual patient.

The introduction of a problem-oriented record dates from 1969[2]. Originally the record was proposed for, and used in medicine, but subsequently its use has been extended to dentistry[3] and optometry[4,5] and examination systems have been devised based on the problem-oriented approach.

This form of routine and documentation is probably suited best to situations in which several examiners have to be responsible for the complete management of the patient as in hospital or clinic.

Base data list

Considerable thought must be given to deciding the information to be gathered for all patients in eye examination — the defined data (*Table 4.1*). The necessity for certain types of information is obvious — symptoms, visual acuities, refraction details — but there would be discussion on others such as colour vision, stereopsis, tonometry, keratometry, balancing methods, and so on. And, how much detail should be obtained on the patient — the 'patient profile'? Apart from the routine information of name, age, sex, occupation, should this also encompass examiner's comments on personality traits, speech, hygiene, habits and other examiner-subjective data? A lone examiner being the only person involved, can readily define the essential information to be collected but, as for conventional printed records, once several examiners become responsible for a system, widely varying opinions have to be reconciled.

Problem-specific data included in the data base consists of those problems reported by the patient and those found by the examiner during examination. Thus, there are *subjective* problems, usually symptoms, such as alleged 'loss' of vision, and *objective* problems, such as depigmented retinal areas seen by ophthalmoscopy.

The problem-oriented system can indicate questions to the examiner as well as to

TABLE 4.1. Defined Data List for Optometric Examination (information to be obtained for every patient)

Patient profile data

Surname	Forenames	Designation	Date and place* of birth
Age	Marital status	Present address	Telephone
Medical practitioner	Present occupation and activities	Recreations	Hobbies

Examiner's general observations, assessments and evaluation*

| Personality* | Motivation* | Behaviour* | Reliability* | Physique* |

History

Optical	Visual	Ocular	Medical
Social*	Occupational	Family	General health
			Present medications

Subjective problems

| Symptoms | Reasons for examination | Other problems |

Present optical corrections in use

| Spectacles | Contact lenses | Uses | Prescriber(s) |
| Date(s) | | | |

Vision

| Patient's opinion* | Assessment with and without prescriptions (if worn) | Distance and near |

Anterior segment and external examination

Facial symmetry	Orbits	Crystalline lens	Near point of
Cover test, distance/near	Motility	Pupillary distance	convergence
Cornea	Adnexa	Conjunctiva	Digital palpation
Pupillary reflexes	Anterior chamber	Iris	Pupils

Posterior segment and internal examination

| Vitreous humour | Fundus (*see Notes*) |

Refraction — objective

Retinoscopy and/or dynamic retinoscopy*, keratometry*, objective optometry*

Refraction — subjective

| Subjective refraction and/or subjective optometry* | Visual acuities | Amplitudes of accommodation* | Near vision additions |

Oculomotor balance

Distance/near

Binocular vision

| Status | Fusion* | Stereopsis* | Fixation disparity* |
| Fusional reserves* Distance/near | | | |

Other data

| Confrontation examination* | Visual field screening* | Colour vision* | Tonometry* |

Prescriptions and lenses advised/prescribed. Uses

Notes
(1) Asterisks indicate areas of investigation on which there may be differences of opinion on the necessity or desirability of inclusion for all patients.
(2) Many items may be subdivided, for example:
    Fundus: colour, pigmentation
    Vessels: pattern, distribution
    Disc: size, colour, shape, vascular distribution, cup/disc ratio, margins, arterial/venous ratio
    Macula
    Periphery
    Fovea: foveal reflex
(3) Minsky's circles[7] with their coded descriptions are useful for recording and identifying media changes at different anteroposterior planes from the corneal epithelium to the posterior vitreous humour.

the patient so that fixed alternative questions may be presented which allow no equivocation: thus:

'Is there cupping of the optic disc?'   Yes/No.

'If so, is it deep, moderate or shallow?'

Forced choice questions of this kind are unattractive to many examiners, yet in clearing the mind of peripheral information they assist in the analysis of signs and provide some measure of uniformity in compiling data for different patients.

The plan of action includes indicated treatment and advice given to the patient. Progress notes identify the standing of each problem at a given time with revised plans for treatment if needed.

The appeal of a problem-oriented approach, as for all record systems, depends on individual preference and attitudes to the eye examination procedures. One advantage is that it concentrates the examiner's attention in a way not possible with conventional recording methods. Any examiner who has had students or colleagues as observers realizes the effect of such bystanders in highlighting weaknesses in technique, understanding and clinical deduction. The comprehensive nature of problem-oriented records demands a similar kind of commitment by the examiner in that all data must be entered in writing. This is demanding in effort and time and the examiner's skills may be dissipated in working the system rather than attending to the patient's real complaints — a paradox in terms of the basic purpose. A supra-abundance of data is self-defeating and the organization of a problem-oriented system and record is a critical exercise if it is to succeed. Nevertheless, the single-handed practitioner can profit from a re-examination of basic routines and recording along problem-oriented lines. For example, on most record cards, the patient's problems, including symptoms, tend to be concealed in the history and symptom abstracts and are not immediately manifest. There is logic in selecting out these subjective problems for emphasis, because the patient expects action to be taken to resolve those problems and for those proposals to be communicated at the end of the examination. Thus, very simply, a patient problem list can be registered on the record thus.

(1) Difficulty in reading
(2) Frontal headaches (with details) } Subjective problems
(3) Low amplitude of accommodation
(4) High physiological exophoria } Objective problems

Complete examples of problem-oriented records are inappropriate here but fuller details may be found in the papers indicated at the end of this chapter.

Computerized clinical data storage and retrieval

The micro-computer has revolutionized many spheres of activity and it has considerable potential in all areas of optometry. Along with the decrease in size of computers has come a progressive reduction in data processing time so that computer-assisted practice management is within reach of even the single-handed practitioner.

Solomons[8], for example, has devised a total optometric practice system run on micro-computer with five modules and several routines covering such practice matters as clinical records, administration, lens stock control, reminder routine, dispensing information, contact lenses, and so on. Special knowledge of computers is not needed.

The present mode of storage of patients' clinical information uses a disc system, the 'floppy' disc which allows a faster recall time than previous data storage methods. The most convenient method of access and input is by conventional keyboard with data on visual display. Extra security can be obtained by the use of 'passwords' which must be known to the computer before entry can be made into any of the stored information.

Like all record systems computerized clinical data storage has disadvantages, but these may be overcome by further research and development.

(1) Because the present mode of access is normally by typewriter keyboard, then some skill in typing is necessary. The speed of input or retrieval of information will be governed by the examiner's prowess in typing. Fowler[9], however, considers that keyboard access could give way to automatic feeding of data to the computer from instruments such as refracting units and that voice recognition systems could be used for the direct storage of patient's problems and history.

(2) With the display of patient's clinical information on standard visual display units there is a possibility that this confidential data could be overseen by others, so that measures must be taken to protect the screen from observation by unauthorized persons.

(3) Machine breakdown results in loss of access.

(4) Floppy discs are best duplicated and these duplicates stored elsewhere than in the practice as a safeguard against damage, loss or against information being accidentally or deliberately wiped out of the system.

(5) The cost of the hardware and software is still relatively high by traditional standards for the individual practitioner.

(6) Computer equipment tends to date rapidly with continuing development.

(7) Availability of updating software and servicing hardware[10] must be considered when purchasing the equipment.

The impact of the micro-computer in optometry is only recently being felt, but the use of sophisticated computer-assisted systems for practice management and particularly for clinical records will depend entirely on the preferences of the individual practitioner.

For further details the references given at the end of the chapter provide additional information on computer assistance in practice.

Computers as a future clinical aid for analysis, evaluation and diagnosis in optometry

The potential of the micro-computer does not cease with practice management and records. Computer systems have already been used as an aid to diagnosis in medicine, and this kind of use should eventually become available in eye examination. The examiner will have access to a wide range of diagnostic information based on the best knowledge and experience of the time with the possibility of constant updating[11]. From an input of individual patient data, recommendations will be available on: other examinations which should be carried out within the capabilities and responsibilities of the examiner; other information which should be solicited from the patient; identifying the causes of problems and symptoms giving a probability ranking, and courses of action open to the examiner.

Other computer-assisted and automatic developments for optometry

Visual display units using colour will allow for the generation of many different forms of test object for use in eye examination. Some of the most useful are: gratings for the investigation of contrast sensitivity; test characters in different shapes, sizes, colours and contrasts; variable saturation colour naming and discrimination tests; pseudo-isochromatic diagrams.

Automatic ophthalmoscopy and external eye examination may become available using variable magnification and video-cassette reproduction with the future possibility of transmitting that and all other patient data for 'telediagnosis'[12], a diagnostic facility which will not require the patient at that time to attend at some distant centre.

These developments have an additional long-term problem in the safeguarding of confidentiality of clinical information and are therefore unlikely to evolve rapidly except in pilot form.

References

1 HURST, J.W. and WALKER, H.K. (1972). *Problem-oriented System.* New York: Medecom Press

2 WEED, L.L. (1969). *Medical Records, Medical Education and Patient Care.* Cleveland: Case Western Reserve University Press

3 TRYON, A.F., MANN, W.V. and DE JONG, N. (1976). 'Use of a problem-oriented dental record in undergraduate dental education.' *J. dent. Educ.,* **40,** 9, 601–608

4 SLOAN, P.G. (1978). 'A problem-oriented optometric record?' *Am. J. Optom. physiol. Optics,* **55,** 5, 352–357

5 BARRESI, B.J. and NYMAN, N.N. (1978). 'Implementation of the problem-oriented system in an optometric teaching clinic.' *Am. J. Optom. physiol. Optics,* **55,** 11, 765–770

6 WICK, R.E. and WICK, B. (1974). 'Clinical recording of fundus features.' *Am. J. Optom. physiol. Optics,* **51,** 3, 214–219

7 MINSKY, H., cited by BERENS, C. (1949). *The Eye and its Diseases,* p. 155 (Ed. by Berens C.). Philadelphia: Saunders

8 SOLOMONS, H. (1980). 'Microprocessors in the consulting room.' *Optician,* **16,** 39–41; **18,** 47–51; **20,** 7–14

9 FOWLER, C.W. (1981). 'Wider uses of the computer in practice.' In *Revolution in the Consulting Room,* **9,** 1–6. Sutton, Surrey: IPC Conferences Ltd.

10 DINNING, J.A. (1981). 'Choosing a microcomputer.' *Ophthal. Opt.,* **21,** 24, 778–780

11 BALL, G.V. (1979). 'Advances in ophthalmic instrumentation.' S.M.C. 350th Anniversary Lecture. *Optician,* **178,** 14–17

12 SHIMAMOTO, S., MATSUBARA, H. and ITOI, M. (1978). 'The fundus camera with an infra-red T.V. system.' *Trans. int. Symp. ophthal. Opt.* (Tokyo), 141–144

Further reading

Revolution in the Consulting Room (1981). *Optician* '81 Conference, Brighton. Sutton, Surrey: IPC Conferences Ltd.

Symposium on Ocular Photodocumentation (1979). *Am. J. Optom physiol. Optics,* 545–604

Chapter 5

Non-tolerance to optical prescriptions

'I can't get on with these glasses . . .'

Grief cases, refraction failure, non-tolerances,[1-4] call them what you will, present some of the most fascinating yet frustrating aspects of optometric practice. No prescriber of optical corrections can be entirely free of occasional failures even where ultra-conservative techniques are practised[5] such as omitting oblique-axis cylinders wherever possible. Some prescribers maintain that they do not have 'grief' cases. Either the problems are dealt with at a different level, for example, by associated staff, or the patients never go back to complain. These latter patients — those who do not return to the original prescriber — are the most problematic because they are an unknown factor. In them, maybe, lies some failure in communication just as the returning belligerent complainer signals a breakdown in practitioner/patient relationship which has to be carefully resurrected.

Most failures are not serious except insomuch as they concern the relationship between patient and practitioner. Nevertheless, because the cause of non-tolerance to a prescription can be as simple and as easily managed as apparent magnification with a recent presbyopic prescription or as urgent as recent detachment of the retina, a planned method of procedure is needed if patients who required some immediate action are to be identified. The actual method employed will vary with the preferences of the examiner but a systematic mode of investigation should always be pursued.

Prescription-induced symptoms

In the course of prescribing optical corrections for eye defects, the hoped-for result is a lasting elimination of the existing symptoms but this is not always realized. Other, less desirable, effects occur.

(1) *Temporary elimination of existing symptoms which then recur* suggests a placebo type effect, with the cause of symptoms remaining unidentified (*see also* (3)).

(2) *Elimination of existing symptoms, replaced by different ones,* is a well-known effect occurring with some commonly prescribed corrections as in corrected presbyopia and fully corrected myopia.

Reading blur is eliminated in *corrected presbyopia* and a comfortable working distance restored. These original symptoms are replaced by apparent magnification and near discomfort often described by the patient as 'pulling' or 'drawing' of the eyes. Usually these are temporary effects which disappear without alteration of the prescription. Sometimes there can be an unintended over-correction of positive power; sometimes, in the higher additions, a need for base in prism.

Distance blur is eliminated in *fully corrected myopia* and replaced by visual discomfort including micropsia; increased contrast and unwanted clarity — usually all temporary.

(3) *Continuation of existing symptoms.* When the need for that type of optical correction is not the underlying cause of symptoms, as in psychoneurosis, then symptoms will be unrelieved (*see also* (1)).

(4) *Continuation of existing symptoms, in a more intense form, often compounded by others previously non-existent,* arises if an optical correction designed to correct ametropia increases an existing heterophoria which itself is the major cause of the patient's symptoms.

(5) *Production of symptoms where none existed previously.* Where no symptoms exist there must be compelling reasons for prescribing as when the lack of good stereopsis resulting from ametropic monocular blur, might be a hazard in the patients occupation. Symptomless astigmatic errors, if corrected, are likely to give rise to apparent distortion of the environment, especially where the axes are oblique.

Some effects are so well known that their cause is easily identifiable, such as the apparent magnification of a recent presbyopic addition. Others baffle the most experienced prescriber. These latter patients, often neurotic in disposition, but sometimes having an undiscovered and unusual optical or other type of abnormality, visit examiner after examiner, collecting marginally different prescriptions and each, after a trial period, giving no greater relief than the last. This type of patient is not common but when such problems do arise, only time and persistence will provide a lasting solution, sometimes needing the involvement of other health professions.

Where unwanted effects arise in prescribing there is a danger of loss of confidence by the patient in the examiner's ability dependent on how well the possible difficulties have been anticipated and explained at an earlier stage. First-time prescriptions, marked changes, introduction of cylindrical elements not worn before — these and other projected alterations in patients' visual habits call for indications by the examiner of possible strangeness with the new prescription. Recording the advice given to the patient is desirable so that they may be reminded of that advice should problems later arise: 'I expect you remember my mentioning that you might find things a little strange for a short time with the new prescription.'

Visual distortion and displacement from optical prescriptions

An extensive literature exists[6] on adaptation to distorted input into the visual system.

It is most likely that after a rapidly acting proprioceptive change, a consolidated visual adaptation takes place. The reality of that adaptation is of the greatest importance to all those who have to prescribe optical corrections for patients. Early workers in modern optometry must have been made regularly aware of initial visual difficulties with some of their prescriptions and, equally, will have noted their disappearance in many patients after a short time. From these and similar experiences it became usual to assume that all such difficulties could be explained in terms of adaptation, personality problems or mistakes in the eye examination process. Conventional wisdom suggested three courses of action: (1) advise the patient that these problems would disappear in a few days; (2) if still unresolved, retain the glasses for a few days and then return them unaltered — a placebo course of action; or (3) assume an 'error' in prescribing and carry out a further eye examination.

These actions are justifiable only where the examiner is satisfied that sufficient information has been obtained about the problems to warrant that course of action. If taken without proper discussion of the patient's problems then a different, but simple, explanation for the difficulties might be overlooked (for example, an error in dispensing) or some condition needing urgent attention (for example, recent detachment of the retina).

Most experienced practitioners develop their own rules and routines for managing the patient who has tolerance problems.

These problems are very varied and may be persistent or only very temporary. The cause can be as diverse as simple dispensing or prescribing errors, mistakes in interpreting written prescriptions, psychoneuroses or recently manifested eye disease. In many cases the cause is obvious after a few questions and answers; in isolated cases a whole range of clinical investigations may be needed before a satisfactory explanation is found, if at all.

Apparent minification of objects and increased contrast are common observations reported by recently corrected myopes. Presbyopic corrections frequently give rise to apparent magnification and discomfort around the eyes. If the practitioner's rapport with the patient has not developed satisfactorily, or problems have not been foreseen, then not only does the patient have discomfort and visual problems, but also dissatisfaction, which may reflect on their judgement of the practitioner's ability. Their attitude can be apologetic and tentative, or aggressive and impolite. Some patients are reluctant to return but quickly adapt and just as rapidly forget the difficulties. Others resort to other prescribers, who may or may not then get in touch with the original examiner.

Most of the distortions produced by common optical prescriptions are overcome in a few days but if the optometrist has failed to anticipate or over-stressed them then the psychological effect on the patient can be damaging both in relation to the prescription and the patient's attitude to the prescriber.

How to anticipate the possible temporary adverse effects of prescriptions without thereby precipitating a psychological non-tolerance is a delicate matter, yet, in prescriptions where the probability is high, some indication to the patient is desirable if only to avoid future loss of confidence. Where the patient already wears a prescription it is always useful to obtain information by indirect questioning on whether the patient remembers ever having had difficulties with new glasses. The answers will condition the way in which possible problems are anticipated to the patient. If there appears to be a long history of non-tolerance, then the nature of those previous problems must be sought and the information found may help avoid a similar occurrence. It may suggest caution in prescribing a full presbyopic addition or the need for special care in deciding the form of bifocal prescription.

Every experienced examiner will have met patients who make the following type of observation: 'I have never been able to wear my last glasses and I'm wearing my old ones.' In this type of patient there is no greater satisfaction than to be able to examine the two prescriptions side by side, lens for lens, power for power, axis for axis, frame for frame, but this is best done alone, free from the distractions and comments of the patient and should always be carried out by the examiner and not by other staff. From these comparisons the reasons for the patient's problem usually become evident. Where they do not, then the patient's description of their troubles must be thoroughly probed if the examiner is to be reasonably sure of not precipitating a similar non-tolerance. However, sometimes a patient must be urged to wear a difficult prescription for its long-term visual effect where, for example, the correction of anisometropia will result in proper binocular and stereoscopic vision for occupational needs.

Patients have come to demand immediate visual satisfaction from optical prescriptions and the examiner who always uses a guarded approach in prescribing reinforces this expectation at the expense of maximizing the visual potential of a proportion of patients. These are the patients who are likely to have tolerance problems and who might need several changes in prescription over a short time. The resulting benefit when visual comfort is obtained is remarkably satisfying to the examiner and to the patient, although it can be very costly. Prescriptions for anisometropia, aphakia, high myopia and large amounts of heterophoria, all may precipitate tolerance problems but it is not the purpose here to deal in depth with dispensing and prescribing for these conditions.

Adverse effects of prescriptions

Prescription-induced symptoms or adverse effects are very varied and in some cases exaggerate the problems which they were designed to alleviate (*Table 5.1*).

Anxiety induced by the examiner

By words and actions the examiner communicates with the patient. Sometimes the expected reaction is opposite to that intended. 'There is nothing at all for you to worry about' said to a patient as reassurance, when referring that patient for other special examinations is just as likely to provoke anxiety as relief. Reassurance should never be given in that over-simple way. It should be done by giving a greater measure of information in an easily understood and honest manner.

It is imprudent to point out the existence of interesting optical or visual phenomena, unknown to the patient and irrelevant to their main problems. It is therefore mischievous to draw the attention of the normal patient to simple phenomena such as physiological diplopia or to muscae unless these effects have previously been reported. The patient may show a passing interest, only to become bedevilled with the phenomenon, developing a neurotic fixation which may take weeks or months to overcome. The prescriber must realize that some forms of clinical comment made in discussion or during eye examination may well cause anxiety. Certain words or phrases should be avoided (*see Table 3.1* on page 16).

Whispered conversations with colleagues beyond a half-closed consulting room office door, even if they do not relate to that patient at all, give rise to morbid fears, especially in older patients. Leaving a patient unattended in the examination room with no explanation for absence is inexcusable, particularly if the examiner re-enters with a colleague clutching an ophthalmoscope. A simple truthful prior explanation helps to avoid distress. The examination record should not be left on view in the absence of the examiner. Most patients are curious about their ills and given that opportunity will take a hurried glance, only to misinterpret or misconstrue, and become even more anxious. Likewise, the examiner must not make plain the intention to cover up or remove the record card if leaving the consulting room. It should be obscured in a discreet, unobtrusive way.

For this reason certain information on the patient is best recorded in an indecipherable shorthand or even in a personal code (for example, suspected but

TABLE 5.1. Prescription-induced Symptoms, Transient or Persistent

Symptom-type	Presenting symptoms	Examples of possible cause (non-pathological)
Referred or sympathetic	Headaches	High presbyopic additions
	Dizziness, giddiness, nausea, disorientation, unreality	Unintended prismatic effects (for example, faulty centration), prismatic corrections (*see also* spatial distortion, below)
Ocular	Discomfort and irritation described variously as 'drawing', 'pulling', 'straining' or 'staring' for 'clear' vision	Recent presbyopic additions
Visual		
Micropsia		Recent myopic prescriptions
		Base out prisms
Macropsia		Recent presbyopic additions
		Base in prisms
General spatial distortions		Unaccustomed cylinders
		Corrected anisometropia
		Change of lens form
Peripheral spatial distortion		Some multifocals
Blurred vision		Inappropriate use of prescription
		Uncorrected residual errors
		Positioning of bifocal segments
		Incorrect effective power of prescription
		Marginally over-corrected positive power resulting from maximum + routine and finite test chart distance
Diplopia		Faulty lens centration
		Improperly corrected astigmatism
		Interference from bifocal segment edge
Chromatopsia		High additions in some fused bifocals
Visual unease		Marginal blur in dominant eye
		Altered muscle balance from previous prescription
Photophobia		Recent contact lenses
		Omission of previously worn tints
Increased contrast		Recently and fully corrected myopia
Unwanted clarity		
'Ghost' images		Reflections from lens surfaces
Other effects		
Lenses feel 'too strong'		Fully corrected myopia and presbyopia
Cosmetic and allied problems		For example, centre or edge thickness of lenses, visibility of bifocal segments, weight of spectacles
Stumbling, tripping		Distorting elements of prescriptions, unaccustomed bifocals

unconfirmed well-known diseases such as tumours, tuberculosis, syphilis). If a code is used then its key should be kept in a known place so that locum tenens examiners can interpret the information or as a safeguard against the failing memory of the examiner.

Causes of non-tolerance

Tables 5.1 and *5.2* summarize some of the common causes of non-tolerance.

Dispensing errors

The most likely explanation to account for a patient's tolerance problem is to be found in the prescription dispensing. All optometrists will be able to quote examples of errors and accidental mistakes, even of the wrong glasses being given out to a patient as a result of the confusion of a common name such as Smith or Jones. Of course, errors should not arise but even the best managed practice is liable to have lapses on occasions, especially in times of pressure or illness. If mistakes occur, then it is imperative to institute a rigorous investigation in an attempt to identify the cause.

Some simple dispensing errors for which the practitioner must always be on the alert[1] include: (1) misreading a badly written prescription, for example, 160 might be misread as 100; (2) errors in transposition and neutralization resulting in a cylinder being 90 degrees off axis; (3) transposition of the prescription for right and left eyes.

Good and regularly appraised practice management is essential to minimizing such disasters.

TABLE 5.2. Some General Causes of Non-tolerance

Practitioner related	Dispensing faults
	Errors in refraction or prescription
	Undetected or subsequently developed eye disease
	Faulty management of initial eye examination
Patient related	Adaptation effects
	Motivation
	Financial problems
Patient/practitioner relationship	Practice environment
	Attitudes and personality patterns of examiner and patient

Refraction and prescribing problems

Common causes of initial prescription problems are: (1) presbyopic addition too large; (2) relative prismatic effects ignored (especially vertical effects); (3) previous lens form significantly changed; (4) effectivity factors overlooked; (5) vocational use not properly determined; (6) slight distance blur due to refraction routine especially in hypermetropic prescriptions.

Table 5.1 indicates the relationship between presenting symptoms and possible cause in both dispensing and refraction anomalies.

Management of initial examination

Well-presented information and advice to the patient will prevent many cases of non-tolerance. It should be a maxim of optometric practice to give every patient a simple explanation for their problems, where this can be determined; and equally a simple statement of the treatment proposed together with advice on possible adverse effects.

The ideal time to devote to an eye examination is debatable and depends on the skill and experience of the examiner. It can be too short, in that the patient feels inadequate attention has been given, but it can also be so long that the patient becomes unduly fatigued and judges the practitioner to be incompetent. Both can precipitate non-tolerance but most likely many of these patients will never return anyway. The optometrist must maintain composure and control of the refraction routine whatever the day-to-day pressures being experienced and adapt the tempo of examination to the particular patient.

Semantic awareness must be kept in mind, particularly when discussing changes of prescription with myopes. Myopic patients are often hypersensitive to increases in their prescription and it is preferable to discuss 'changes' in prescription rather than use words such as 'stronger' (*see* Chapter 3).

Patient-orientated aetiology and relationships

Patient psychology and relationships present the most difficult, but challenging, area for managing non-tolerance. Interesting papers and texts have appeared on the general question of psychosomatic phenomena related to the eye[7,8] and on the personality pattern of the patient.

The milder psychotic states can be ocular-related and placebo-type treatment, such as the temporary correction of minor refractive errors may help the patient but these must be prescribed with caution (*see* Placebos in optometry, page 44).

Many questionnaire-type systems have been developed for assessing personality variables but these are mostly research-orientated and not designed for the consulting room or optometric office. The description of symptoms by the patient provides an indication of the emotional state. One patient will appear to be entirely incapacitated and develop a description in florid terms. This applies particularly to eye-related sympathetic symptoms such as headaches. Another, more stable, individual with the same disability will present a coherent and logical analysis, leading directly to a diagnosis.

Investigation and management of non-tolerance

Optometrists have a basic routine for eye examination which is adaptable to the particular patient. There should also be an equally adaptable routine of investigation for patients who have problems with prescriptions from whatever cause. Nothing is more damaging to the practitioner than to appear to be irritated by such patients. Nothing can be so rewarding as to find a valid explanation for a patient's symptoms, but nothing can be so frustrating as to fail to explain the problems even after the most careful examination. A planned and controlled management routine can lessen the likelihood of the latter occurring. In all health sciences which deal individually with patients, including optometry, it is sound practice to listen to the patient's description of their symptoms and history and, if the aetiology is obscure, to exclude the simpler causes before considering others. The most important first steps in non-tolerance examination, therefore, accords with this philosophy. The problems must be discussed fully and then the prescription and dispensing aspects must be checked in detail. It is important to verify the prescription against the original examination record and for the optometrist to hold these discussions in the private, confidential atmosphere of the consulting room.

Suggested check list routine for tolerance problems

(1) *Listen to and record fully the patients complaints.* Encourage the patient to elaborate freely on all aspects of their problems.

(2) *Check dispensing aspects.* Verify the prescription against the optometrist's initial examination. Check accuracy, lens type, relative prismatic effects, base curves,

tints, possible lens faults. Frame type, colour and fit must also be considered. If no obvious cause is disclosed then adopt the following.

(3) *Compare vision with the new prescription to the visual acuity previously recorded, binocular and monocular.* Demonstrate vision with the new prescription before that of any previous prescription. This avoids a patient realizing that their old prescription gives worse vision than the new one and in some cases, rapidly adapting their description of vision with the new prescription to suit their complaint.

(4) *Consider previous advice.* Has the advice been followed? For example, is the patient using the prescription incorrectly? It is not unknown for a patient to be wearing reading glasses out of doors or expecting to see clearly across a room with that prescription.

(5) *Consider the change from the previous prescription.* This may have been too great for adaptation to take place rapidly. Patients, especially older ones, who have not changed their glasses for many years may be found to need a considerable increase in distance positive power which will not be tolerated easily at first, especially when compounded into an increased presbyopic addition.

(6) *Consider developed abnormality, or previously undetected conditions.* (1) and (3) may indicate such possibilities. The presence or absence of symptoms without the prescription is, of course, most significant. Recent retinal detachment and chronic angle closure glaucoma are notable conditions to consider.

(7) *Consider patient psychology.* (*a*) Neurosis such as hypochondria, obsessional or anxiety states; (*b*) motivation, for example, adverse reaction to wearing glasses, displeasure with some dispensing aspect, financial problems.

(8) *Check refraction as indicated by (1), (3) and (5).* Attention to related ocular functions such as disturbed muscle balance, and fixation disparity.

Placebos in optometry

A placebo is defined in medicine as an inert substance given to please a patient, the word being derived from the Greek meaning 'to please'. In optometry, placebos can be real optical prescriptions or they are just as likely to be psychological gambits used deliberately, or unconsciously, by the examiner.

The conscientious practitioner often hears the following type of comment from a quite ordinary patient after a quite uneventful eye examination using no more than traditional methods. 'I have never had such a thorough examination.'

The patient is pleased and impressed with the examination and with the attention received. Confidence has been generated in the examiner, in the techniques used and indirectly in the results obtained, and in the decisions being made. On those psychological grounds alone the patient may be less liable to experience and report problems with a potential problem-precipitating prescription. A complex examination technique using complex-looking apparatus or an examination which appears to be exacting and detailed, based on the patient's previous experience, acts as a placebo to some susceptible individuals. The red-green lights of bichromatic tests, the curious visual effects produced by polarized dissociation, the flashing lights of field screeners or the futuristic design of some consulting room instrument ensembles — all contribute placebo-like additions in some patients, particularly those who can recollect more spartan examinations.

Placebos in optometry can, however, be very direct, akin to the inert substances sometimes used in medical treatment. Small optical prescriptions for minor degrees of hypermetropia or for with and against the rule astigmatism must often rate as placebos, and expensive ones at that. Sometimes small prescriptions are given as a 'trial' by an examiner having to make a forced choice decision at the end of an examination in order to avoid equivocation in front of the patient. The optometric and related literature contains examples of optical prescribing technique and dogma which are suggestive of a placebo effect, although in an *ex post facto* situation it is difficult to establish this with certainty. The relief of symptoms on correcting small amounts of astigmatism as low as 0.12 D[9], very small base in prisms as a relief for migraine headache[10], the prismatic correction of minor degrees of horizontal heterophoria or the use of mildly tinted lenses may all rank as optical placebos on many occasions. This is not to condemn all small optical prescriptions nor their occasional use as placebos. Small oblique astigmatism and low myopia, when corrected, significantly raise vision especially for occupational purposes. Placebo-type actions of many different forms, including lenses, seem to help some patients at a stressful and anxiety-laden period of their lives where proper counselling is unavailable or has been rejected. These patients present referred symptoms of eye discomfort and headaches, and an optical placebo may help overcome immediate problems but should then be discarded.

This can be a costly procedure in terms of skilled time and patient finance, but it is no more or no less ethical than all placebo procedures provided that its justification is based on sound principles or proven experience. The danger exists that a prescription given for its temporary effect will become a permanent crutch for that patient. All experienced examiners will have met patients who have lost or broken their only spectacles and who appear to be under considerable stress. On examination the prescription appears to be negligible, well within normally expected tolerance limits. It is reasonable to suppose, therefore, that some small optical prescriptions, particularly small positive lenses given to young persons at moments of life stress, have become permanent psychological additions to their lives, fearful of unleashing those original symptoms if the lenses are discarded.

The optical effect of low positive over-corrections in young people (for example, R and L + 0.50 D) prescribed for near work is to soften the outlines of distant objects when the patient looks through these lenses into the distance, as they invariably will on occasion. A sharp image to the visual environment emphasizes cold reality. In the softer world of a positive over-correction facial expressions are less discernible, blurred objects appear more distant and the individual is more able to retreat from involvement.

These prescribing situations and the significance in them of the placebo effect have received little attention in optometry. Detailed studies are needed to identify the patients in which their use is justifiable and to clarify what elements in those prescribing situations and in what measure contribute in placebo terms. Discussion of problems and advice is much preferable if time is available and the practitioner will often become involved with patients in a counselling capacity.

Until more reliable information becomes available, the prescribing of placebos in the form of optical prescriptions should be infrequent and even then only with extreme care.

References

1 BALL, G.V. (1977). 'Unverträglichkeit gegenüber optischen Verordnungen.' *Trans. int. Opt. Kong.*, pp. 41–48. Düsseldorf

2 BELMONT, O (1961). 'Refraction troubles.' *Int. ophthal. Clin.,* **1,** 261–275
3 GILKES, M.J. (1966). 'Problems in refraction.' *Trans. ophthal. Soc. U.K.,* **86,** 657–666
4 STANWORTH, A. (1966). 'Refraction failures.' *Trans. ophthal. Soc. U.K.,* **86,** 677–698
5 CARTER, DARRELL, B. (Ed) (1967). 'Symposium on conventional wisdom in optometry.' *Am. J. Optom.,* **44,** 11, 731–745
6 KOHLER, I. (1964). *The Formation and Transformation of the Perceptual World* (trans. H. Fiss). New York: International Universities Press
7 DREWS, R.C. (1967). 'Organic versus functional ocular problems.' *Int. ophthal. Clin.,* **7,** 665–696
8 SCHLAEGEL, T.F. and HOYT, W.F. (1957). *Psychosomatic Ophthalmology.* Baltimore: Williams & Wilkins
9 GILES, G.H. (1960). *The Principles and Practice of Refraction,* p. 286. London: Hammond Hammond
10 TURVILLE, A.E. (1934). 'Refraction and migraine.' *Br. J. physiol. Opt.,* **8,** 62–89

Further reading

CORNSWEET, T.N. (1970). *Visual Perception.* New York: Academic Press
KOHLER, I. (1964). *The Formation and Transformation of the Perceptual World* (trans. H. Fiss). New York: International Universities Press
ROCK, I. (1966). *The Nature of Perceptual Adaptation.* New York: Basic Books

Part II

Problem-specific data arising from the history and symptom interview — analysis

Chapter 6

Visual blur — 'loss' of vision and visual unease

'I don't seem to recognize people across the road as well as I used to'.
'I've suddenly noticed that I can't see out of this eye.'

The presenting symptoms of visual blur (*Tables 6.1* and *6.2*) and visual loss are considered together for a number of reasons. First, patients often talk about loss of vision or 'can't see' when their vision is only blurred. Visual acuity may be quite normal with a proper and sometimes quite minor optical correction. Secondly, apparent blurring of vision can be a symptom preceding a real loss of function unless some correcting action is taken. Finally, there may be areas of total visual loss and

TABLE 6.1. Some Causes of the Complaint of Blurred Vision

Uncorrected and poorly corrected ametropia and presbyopia
Defects in spectacle lenses
Accommodation/convergence anomalies
Clinical emmetropia with prolonged close work (distance blur)
Migraine
Primary anomalies of the ocular media, for example, nuclear cataract, vitreous haze, irregularity of
     refracting surfaces
Other conditions which decrease the transparency of the ocular media, for example, posterior uveitis
Central retinal oedema, for example, from commotio retinae
Angle closure glaucoma
Nutritional amblyopia
Uncommon syndromes, for example, Posner–Sclossmann[9]

(*See also* Transient blurring — *Table 6.2*)

areas of reduced function in the same eye. Whichever happens to be nearest to the fixation point usually determines the patient's complaint. However, when a normal eye's perceptual image is fused with a fellow image containing defective areas, visual symptoms of loss of function may be absent in photopic conditions. Under special conditions such as reduced illumination or momentary occlusion of the good eye, these visually deficient areas are likely to become evident to the patient.

Blurred vision

With the possible exception of headaches, blurred vision at some distance or at some time is the most common symptom with which patients present themselves for eye examination. The cause may be as simple as the transient blurring produced by mucus

TABLE 6.2. Some Possible Causes for the Presenting Symptoms of Transient Blurring of Vision Either at Distance or Near

Mucus passing over cornea
Excess lacrimation (*see* Watering eyes on page 114)
Migraine (*see* Photopsia on page 96)
Vitreous opacities or muscae (*see* Entoptic phenomenon on page 99)

Variable spasm of accommodation
- Convergence excess
- Psychoneuroses
- Irritation of ciliary muscle
- Trauma
- Toxins and drugs
- Irritative IIIrd nerve lesions

Variable insufficiency of accommodation
- Early presbyopia or lens sclerosis
- Pseudo-myopia
- Chronic open angle and chronic angle closure glaucoma
- Drugs and toxins
  - Stimulants
  - Tranquillizers
  - Alcohol
  - Diphtheric
- Trauma
- Diabetes and other general medical conditions
- IIIrd nerve lesions

Chronic angle closure glaucoma
Variation in refraction (as in diabetes)
Multiple sclerosis
Functional
Malingering

Note: Where transient blurring of vision is given in the history and not evident at the time of examination then the blurring complained of may have been a real loss of vision, usually central.

passing across the cornea or uncorrected refractive errors, but could also be much more serious such as posterior uveitis or carotid artery insufficiency. The responsibility of the practitioner in examining such patients is evident, but whatever the multitude of possibilities giving rise to the symptom of visual blur, the examiner must always have in mind some idea of relative probability. In general ophthalmic practice having a random patient distribution, blurred vision from a condition such as angle closure glaucoma has a low incidence contrasted, for example, with visual blur due to uncorrected simple myopia. Suspicions of some low incidence condition must be reasonable and based on reasonable evidence, otherwise a very high proportion of all patients with this presenting symptom would be sent for further special investigations following their first visit.

High incidence causes for the presenting symptom of visual blur

Some very simple explanations exist for the symptom of blurred vision, even in quite normal patients. Unless the cause is manifest, the practitioner must first be satisfied that no such simple explanation can account for the presenting symptom.

(1) Patients who have normal visual acuity sometimes complain of blurring when, simply, they have compared their own vision with that of a relative or friend who has supra-normal vision. The comparison arises from activities which demand high visual resolution or where hyper-visual acuity is an advantage. Such activities include reading lettering on distant signposts and advertisement hoardings or, perhaps, the time on a clock tower seen far off. Young people may have visual acuity of the order of 6/4 (20/13) or very rarely as high as 6/3 (20/10). In comparison, a person of the same age with normal visual acuity (6/6) (20/20) will appear to be deficient. The

complainant usually has a minor optical error which needs no correction, often astigmatism at an oblique axis as low as 0.25 D. The patient is mildly alarmed by such findings and reassurance is received with genuine relief.

This kind of patient is frequently supra-conscious of health problems. If the patient is marginally myopic but not at that time requiring correction it may signal the onset of a greater degree of myopia with time and this possibility may be assessed by other signs and symptoms including family history and age of the patient.

(2) Normal patients comment on, rather than complain, that vision indoors becomes blurred when they are tired. The most common reason for this is relaxation of accommodation so that close objects appear blurred. Accompanying this slight blur is a relaxation of convergence. Vision not only becomes blurred but confused due to the transient near diplopia. On being brought back to full consciousness vision immediately becomes clear again. Unusual demands on accommodation as in uncorrected hypermetropia or early presbyopia give rise to similar symptoms and will be determined during eye examination.

(3) Scratches on the front surfaces of spectacle lenses are a common enough reason for visual blur, particularly in presbyopes who are not able to see the lens surfaces clearly when their glasses are removed. Often the patient feels that their spectacle lenses are dirty and reports having tried to clean them but with no improvement. These scratches are caused during work or by regularly placing meniscus or toric lenses with their convex surfaces downwards. A defective area develops in the centre of the front surface of each lens.

(4) Mucus in the conjunctival sac gives a transient visual blur as it passes across the cornea. Mucus organizes under the lids in hay fever sufferers and in mild conjunctivitis or similar conditions and moves when the eye is rubbed. Gross irritation is felt if the mucus has hardened into 'strings' (this is particularly so in hay fever), but if soft, there is little sense of discomfort. Vision becomes momentarily blurred but clears by blinking. Repeated instances of blurring from this cause may alarm the patient. Advice should be directed to relieving the causal condition.

(5) *Excess lacrimal fluid in the conjunctival sac.* Through over-production of tears as on windy days or in emotive situations, tear fluid accumulates in the conjunctival sac and interferes with vision, giving blur and metamorphopsia from the prismatic effect. Blinking removes the blur for a time. The condition is usually apparent to the patient who remarks spontaneously about the effect of wind or dust and their watery eyes under those conditions. Abnormalities of lacrimal secretion or drainage must be investigated. These symptoms tend to occur mainly in older patients in so far as the chronic watery eye is concerned.

Optical causes of blurred vision

Unless there is some special reason for suspecting a non-optical cause for the complaint of blurred vision then the various refractive reasons should first be investigated and excluded.

The patient must amplify the problem in terms of criteria such as onset, duration, progress, variability, and so on. The types of problem-oriented question to be used are similar to those for visual loss (page 54). The symptom of blurred vision resulting from ametropia will be conditioned both by the personality of the patient and by the type of work being undertaken. Outdoor workers can exist with a fairly high degree of hypermetropia without correction and without symptoms until well over the age of 30 years but may be detected earlier through screening programmes. Hypersensitive individuals employed in a visual task such as draughtsmanship may complain of blur which, to the practitioner, is quite minimal — the blur produced, for example, by 0.25 D of bilateral astigmatism even with principal meridians around 180 or 90.

Early myopia

A common complaint in commencing myopia is that distance vision is blurred after close work and takes a little time to become 'clear' again. Students find an annoying latent period for vision of lecture boards to clear after writing notes. Along with slight constant visual blur (the usual symptom), a problem involving re-focusing from near to distance is one indicator to early myopia of the order of 0.50 D or less. Slight spasm of accommodation must be excluded by the usual methods of examination.

Blurred vision in poor illumination

Some uncommon anomalies cause a real elevation in the terminal light threshold (*see* Chapter 9) but, occasionally, corrected myopes notice visual blur or complain of poor vision as the light begins to fail at dusk and before significant photopic symptoms arise. Myopes needing a minor change in their photopic optical prescription are particularly sensitive to this mesopic blur, especially in driving. Emmetropes or other corrected ametropes occasionally experience the same problem. The dilating pupil together with other reasons for the normal low luminance myopic shift of refraction causes slight visual blur.

Related states

Blurred vision occurs as a consequence of anomalies of convergence. In convergence insufficiency, the excessive convergence innovation necessary to retain single vision may produce a spastic and variable state of accommodation which results in distance visual blur. Problems can also result from divergence excess and in any condition which causes spasm of accommodation.

Blurred vision — non-refractive causes

Anything which affects the transparency of the ocular media is liable to precipitate the symptom of visual blur. The conditions are legion and will not be dealt with here in detail except to note some which are of distinct concern to the optometrist and to include some points which are not emphasized in standard texts.

Angle closure glaucoma

The corneal oedema of angle closure glaucoma results not only in the symptom of visual blur being a possible presenting symptom but also in the classic symptom of coloured haloes around white lights (*see* Chapter 10).

Visual blur may sometimes also arise in near work due to reducing accommodation and the positive lens addition needed for comfortable reading would then be in excess of that normally expected for the patient's age. The blur may be accentuated by changes in the crystalline lens. A real reduction in visual acuity will occur in the later stages if the condition remains untreated. However, the incidence of this form of glaucoma and hence the frequency with which it could be expected in the average optometric practice must be considered (Chapter 10). Patients describe their visual experiences in a variety of ways in the early stages of the disease using terms such as cloudiness, mistiness, smokiness, haziness.

Other symptoms typical of angle closure glaucoma occur and would heighten suspicions as, for example, frontal headaches and 'fullness' sensations referred to the eyes often with the failing light at the end of the day.

Open angle glaucoma

If blurring is reported at all in open angle glaucoma it is likely to be an appreciation at a late stage of some loss or extensive reduction of function in part of the visual field, but even this is unusual. Only if the loss approaches the point of fixation is it usually noticed and rarely with binocular vision if the equivalent area of the other eye's visual field is unaffected. However, this type of defect is much more noticeable under reduced illumination and any complaint of blur, loss or difficulty at low luminance levels must be investigated.

Reduced accommodational power may give rise to near blur earlier than warranted by the patient's age and hence the need for a presbyopic addition at that earlier age, higher than usual.

Vitreous haze

The vitreous humour is commonly the site of diffuse-like opacities. These settle by gravity during sleep but, when the patient is active are disturbed so that vision deteriorates during the day. The visual blur is variable. Vitreous haze occurs in the early stages of degenerations of the vitreous humour and in early cyclitis. Variations in vision occur as the patient reads a test chart. At one moment the vitreous particles settle but are stirred up again on the next eye movement.

Loss of vision

Alleged loss of vision will be reported in a variety of ways by patients in answer to an initial open-ended history/symptom question. 'I suddenly noticed that I couldn't see out of my (left) eye.' 'Everything went black for a few seconds.' 'When I close my (left) eye I can't see anything clearly.' 'I've lost the vision in my (left) eye.'

Because the symptom of 'loss' of vision can have so wide an interpretation depending on the particular patient, it can never be treated lightly, even if the practitioner suspects a trivial cause at an early stage. A previously unnoticed amblyopic eye or a unilateral refractive error may precipitate the complaint, but it could also arise from multiple sclerosis or vascular catastrophe.

The first reaction of the examiner must be to probe the patient's choice of words and the meanings attributed to them. What is meant by 'loss'; what is meant by 'left' — Is it left side or left eye? Is vision blurred rather than lost? Is central vision lost or peripheral vision?

It is useful to check the patient's vision at that stage by simple means even if this means deviating from the history/symptom discussion along lines such as 'You feel that you have lost the vision of your left eye . . . do you see anything at all?' 'If I cover off your other eye . . do you see me . . . (if not) do you see anything in the surroundings . . . out of the corner of your eye? (if yes, but blurred) 'Can you recognize the colours of the clothes I am wearing?' 'Can you describe the colour of my suit/dress?' 'What do you see out of the window?' (The uncovered eye should be observed for pendular movements which may indicate a central scotoma.)

These immediate observations are useful in checking whether there appears to be a true loss of function or an acute or long-standing condition causing visual blur. They also indicate whether the defect is right or left hemianopic rather than right or left eyes. The history/symptom interview then continues with problem-oriented questions on aspects of the failure of vision which have not been covered by the patient's initial answers. The information needed is as follows.

(1) Date of onset 'When did you first notice the problem?'

(2) Mode of onset 'Did it seem to occur suddenly or gradually?'

(3) Permanent or transient 'Has it remained the same or varied?'

(4) Activity or event-related 'Do you remember whether you were involved in any particular activity at the time?'

(5) Total or partial 'Do you seem to see anything at all with that eye?'

(6) Unilateral or bilateral (*Tables 6.3, 6.4 and 6.5*) 'Does it seem to affect both or only one eye?' The answer to this question will be the patient's opinion but, as previously noted, 'right' and 'left' eyes may be the description used by patients who have hemianopic-type losses.

TABLE 6.3. True, Sudden, Total, Unilateral Visual Loss

Haemorrhage into the vitreous humour
Occlusion of central retinal artery
Retinal detachment (occurring overnight, it may appear to have been sudden)
Trauma
Acute glaucoma
Functional

(*See also* 'Central' visual loss below)

Note: Sudden central visual loss may be reported as *total* by the patient as in haemorrhage at the macula or in retrobulbar neuritis.

TABLE 6.4. Possible Causes of Bilateral Loss of Central Vision

Migraine (paracentral)
Toxins and drugs (for example, methanol, chronic ethyl alcoholism, lead, etc.)
Macular degeneration
'Eclipse' blindness
Bilateral central retinal oedema
Retrobulbar neuritis, bilateral
Trauma
Nutritional amblyopia
Cortical lesions

TABLE 6.5. Unilateral Loss of Central Vision — Some Conditions

Vitreous opacity
Optic neuritis, acute axial neuritis, retrobulbar neuritis
Macular degeneration or haemorrhage
Central choroiditis
Commotio retinae and other trauma

(7) With or without pain 'Do you recollect whether your eye or around your eyes was painful at the time?'

(8) Previous attacks 'Can you remember ever suffering from anything like this before?'

(9) Other symptoms 'Were you conscious of anything else affecting your eyes or vision at that time?' (Examples may be given if desired).

In unilateral conditions of visual loss with no pain the possibility exists of patients being unaware of their defect for a considerable time. The patient is as likely or as unlikely to notice sudden loss of central vision in *one eye* (for example, unilateral central scotoma) as a total loss of vision in that eye whereas to the practitioner the difference between *total* and *central* loss is highly significant in terms of aetiology. In loss of central vision in both eyes, as in some cases of advanced macular degeneration, the patient will not be able to read, but peripheral vision will allow many activities to be carried out without special training. Patients with bilateral central scotomata which are absolute will be grossly handicapped for any tasks demanding good visual acuity, and the condition and thus the presenting symptoms will be quite apparent to the patient as soon as the scotomata are dense enough for binocular visual acuity to be significantly decreased.

Loss of central vision may be clearly differentiated into categories such as unilateral, absolute, transient, and so on, but there is no equivalent demarcation in the causal factors. Some conditions cause unique defects, others manifest themselves in a variety of ways. Neurological and ophthalmological texts dealing with anomalies of the central field of vision cover individual abnormalities in detail.

In unilateral conditions the good eye's central field overrides that of the affected eye but the loss of the central fusion stimulus may give some sensation of visual unreality and discomfort, especially where there is significant heterophoria. In transient bilateral scotomata the visual acuity may have returned to normal by the time the patient attends for examination. The history and symptom interview will be of great importance in attempting to uncover the state of vision during the 'attack' and in providing indicators for special emphasis during subsequent clinical examinations. Nevertheless, where the symptom is transient and not evident at the time of examination it is often difficult to determine from the patient's account whether the loss was a true one or momentary blur from some cause.

At the simplest level mucus causes irregularity in the retinal image as it crosses the pupil and the patient is likely to report distortion, blur or loss of vision dependent on his or her observation, interpretation and choice of words. At a much more serious level the symptom could result from early multiple sclerosis (*see* below). It is vital therefore to extract as much information as possible from the patient by presenting problem-oriented questions which are later rephrased on a check-recheck basis.

Transient loss of vision with transient diplopia

The retrobulbar neuritis of early multiple sclerosis involves symptoms of transient visual loss. Transient diplopia is another common experience. With remission the symptoms may have disappeared by the time the patient attends for examination. Any complaint of transient visual loss with occasional double vision must be regarded with suspicion and must alert the practitioner to the possibility of these presenting symptoms being an early indicator of multiple sclerosis.

Stress and physical exercise have both been reported to lead to impaired vision as a transient phenomenon in multiple sclerosis[1]. The effect of exercise in raising body temperature is probably the significant factor[2].

Note
With true, sudden, total, bilateral loss of vision as in uraemia, for example, the

TABLE 6.6. Possible Causes of Transient Loss of Vision—Total or Partial

Mucus passing over the cornea (as in hay fever)
Excess lacrimation
Gravitational effects (as in stooping and rising rapidly)
Migraine
Vitreous opacities
Retinal vascular disease, including embolic and spastic episodes
Chronic angle closure glaucoma
Interference of blood supply to optic nerve (for example, raised I.O.P.)
Hypotension (fundal, as in papilloedema)
Vascular insufficiency (for example, carotid artery syndrome)
Optic neuritis, retrobulbar neuritis (as in multiple sclerosis)
Trauma, such as a blow on the eye
General systemic conditions[8] (for example, hypertension)
Functional
Malingering

(*See also* Blurring on page 50)

Note: Where transient loss of vision is given in the history, and not evident at the time of examination,
then the 'loss' may have been incomplete or there may have been visual blur only.

patient will not be brought to the optometrist in general practice unless there is some
most unusual circumstance. This kind of patient may occasionally be seen in clinical
discussions by optometrists associated with hospital practice.

Sudden total unilateral visual loss

If it can be demonstrated that vision has been totally lost in one eye and the onset
appears to have been sudden rather than a previously unnoticed long-standing
condition then one of a number of causes of which this is characteristic will be present
but in general optometric practice having a random catchment, such conditions will
be of low incidence. The task will be to confirm the real loss of vision by the usual
methods of examination, determine whether treatment is already being received and
to record sufficient and relevant details for a subsequent report. The patient will then
be dealt with in accordance with the custom or rules governing practice in the
particular country or state. For example, in the United Kingdom such patients would
be referred to a registered medical practitioner, preferably the one with whom the
patient is registered. Where attention is needed urgently, as in sudden painless visual
loss in one eye, then referral could be direct to the medical personnel in hospital.

    There are many other and varied causes of sudden or partial loss of vision. The
differential diagnosis may take many special investigations outside the sphere of
general optometry but the optometrist will report the significant findings in referring
the patient.

    Where loss of vision is associated with considerable pain and other obvious
symptoms, as in acute glaucoma, then the patient may be prostrated and medical, as
opposed to optometric, attention will have been summoned. In primary health care
these patients would not reach the optometrist unless special circumstances exist such
as geographical isolation. Emergency treatment would then be needed prior to the
patient being transferred for special attention in hospital or clinic.

Loss of peripheral vision

Real loss of peripheral vision occurs in many conditions (*Table 6.7*) but there are

TABLE 6.7. Total or Partial Loss of Peripheral Vision

Migraine (transient and partial)
Glaucoma, especially open angle, later stages
Toxic amblyopia (for example, quinine, chloroquine, arsenic, carbon monoxide)
Retinitis pigmentosa and its variants
Peripheral choroiditis
Chiasmal lesions such as bitemporal hemianopia and its variants
Retrochiasmal lesions, such as homonymous hemianopia and its variants
Trauma (for example, to occipital lobe as in double homonymous hemianopia with macular sparing)
Some forms of optic atrophy (for example, tabetic)
Bilateral occlusion of the central retinal arteries with cilio-retinal central retention (unusual)
Hysteria

several spurious causes in which the patient may report a loss and which may take the practitioner into several time-consuming examination techniques unless careful analysis of the symptoms has been carried out in discussion with the patient (*Table 6.8*). 'I seem to have lost my vision on this side' can suggest any lesion giving homonymous or heteronymous hemianopia, widespread retinal or choroidal degeneration, retinal detachment, the classic problem of advanced open angle glaucoma, retinitis pigmentosa, or merely a faulty spectacle lens or change in postural habits (*Table 6.8*). Patients may complain about colliding with objects or people but this report need not indicate a true peripheral loss. With age a stooping gait is acquired; the general direction of gaze lowered and some restriction of upward gaze occurs[3]. It is quite common for such patients to find themselves hitting overhanging branches of trees with their heads which would have been seen with a more upright posture (*see* below).

TABLE 6.8. Apparent Partial Loss of Peripheral Vision

Spectacle frames, lens faults
Change in postural habits: headwear, hairstyle
High prescriptions, as in aphakia
Environmental factors, especially in performing special visual tasks
Acquired ptosis
Malingering
Miosis

Patients who have lost most of their photopic or scotopic peripheral vision will be quite incapacitated in those conditions, and will need help to get about. Failing to appreciate objects or people on a certain side may indicate hemianopia involving that part of the binocular field. Difficulty in reading accompanied by loss of peripheral vision points to right homonymous hemianopia. Problems in vision in dim illumination arise from senile cortical cataract which reduces retinal illumination and causes irregularities in the retinal image. It can also result from the need for a change in prescription or in the classic case of advanced retinitis pigmentosa (*see* Chapter 9). However, the practitioner must be alert to making assumptions without adequate discussion and examination. Failing to see objects approaching from a certain direction may be due to some quirk of the environment, especially if the patient is involved in a demanding visual task. 'I didn't see him coming' is a common observation after a minor automobile accident. Visual field loss is unlikely. Better to consider inattention, blockage by the internal structures of the automobile or externally in the environment, the effect of spectacle frames, weather conditions or the colour of the approaching vehicle or person in contrast to the surroundings.

Colliding with objects or people

This classic symptom of some form of major visual field defect should not obscure the possibility of a simpler explanation which may be disclosed by detailed discussion of the patient's problem. It has already been pointed out that an older patient may complain of colliding with branches of garden trees and other projections. Hastening to carry out a full visual field examination the examiner finds everything apparently normal. The reason for this can be quite simple. With increasing age many people become bowed from the waist so that the head becomes more and more depressed. The brow and lids then become more effective in reducing vision above the horizontal. Even simpler explanations are possible — the patient has taken to wearing a new type of hat, or has a new frame to distance lenses, even has a new hair style. In visual field examination the head is forced into a more upright position by the forehead rest, where used, and the visual effect of an ageing head posture is obscured.

If a true visual field defect exists sufficient to cause the patient to collide with large objects then confrontation examination should readily demonstrate the loss.

Visual unease

Visual unease will not be described as such in standard works covering eye-related symptoms. It must be distinguished from discomfort in and around the eyes (an ocular rather than a visual symptom) and is a symptom recognized by all those experienced in eye examination.

The patient complains about vision but is unable to give precise indicators to their visual problem. A typical patient gives the following kind of information in the history and symptom interview.

'When I look at things my vision seems to bother me.'

'In what way — can you explain?'

'It's difficult, I seem to have to concentrate to see things properly.'

'Does your vision seem clear in the distance?'

'Yes, it's not blurred or anything like that.'

'And is it clear at near distances, such as in reading?'

'Yes, quite all right.'

'Do you notice the problem all the time?'

'No, not all the time, only every so often.'

'How often — can you say?'

'Oh, several times a day I think.'

'Does it seem to come on mostly when you are out of doors or inside?'

'Mostly inside I think, but I couldn't be definite.'

Sensing the uncertainty an earlier question is re-phrased.

'If you think very carefully about what you see when your vision seems to trouble you, is there anything you notice particularly?'

'Well, I feel as if I'm having to stare at things very hard; I'm having to peer at them to take everything in.'

There could be a communication problem; the patient could be unobservant or merely dull but this type of vague visual complaint is met in patients who have identifiable eye conditions or there may be psychological or neurological problems.

Causes of visual unease *(Table 6.9)*

Ametropia and binocular vision problems

In its simpler forms, visual unease is found in patients who have minor degrees of unilateral uncorrected ametropia and who do not notice that vision using one eye is marginally blurred under certain conditions. Binocular visual acuity is normal.

TABLE 6.9. Some Causes of the Presenting Symptom of Visual Unease

Mucus passing over the cornea
Need for change in optical prescription, often unilateral
Uncorrected ametropia, usually minor and unilateral
Minor stresses in binocular fusion or accommodation
Effect of drugs and toxins
Loss of contrast sensitivity (demyelinating disease, glaucoma, diabetes)
Epilepsy
Neurological lesions
Psychological disorders

The sense of ill-defined strangeness probably arises when the 'good' eye becomes occluded momentarily through some obstruction in the environment. The transient blur does not register and is not a presenting symptom but reaches consciousness only as a sense of mild visual discomfort.

The need for a change in prescription in corrected ametropes commonly gives this kind of symptom also. A patient comments: 'I don't feel comfortable with my glasses.' Although there could be several causes it is common to find slight distance or near blur in one eye, not appreciated as such by the patient. The complaint of having to concentrate on or stare at objects often arises if accommodation is just being overtaxed as in uncorrected hypermetropia or in the need for a low presbyopic addition. The later examination confirms these states.

Fleeting unreality in the environment can also arise as a result of stress in binocular fusion attributable to transient unilateral central suspension (a somewhat similar) problem occurs in the use of a mirror septum when patients remark that the patch on the mirror 'bothers' them). The usual methods for investigating the quality of binocular vision, fusion and heterophoria will determine the anomaly. It is useful also to question the patient about binocular vision in low illumination as in night driving. Fusional stress, compensated in photopic conditions, demonstrates itself as annoying transient diplopia for small bright light sources in mesopic and scotopic conditions. The high relative luminance of these sources contrasted with the background and the absence of substantial peripheral fusional elements makes suspension more difficult hence the transient diplopia.

Psychological and neurological problems

Psychological and neurological disorders give visual symptoms varying from a mere feeling of unease or unreality to gross changes of visual perception (*see also* Hallucinations, Chapter 10).

Patients who experience bizarre disorders of vision rarely consult the optometrist in the first instance and, if they do, the symptom discussion rapidly discloses the extreme nature of the presenting symptoms such as fragmentation of the perceptual visual environment or palinopsia (*see* below). Uncomplicated ametropia or binocular vision anomalies do not precipitate symptoms of this order.

The optometrist is more likely to examine patients suffering eye and visual problems arising from mild psychotic states as in stress and anxiety, and in these states complaints about vision and eyes are common[4]. Colourful or stressful analogies may be made in describing their visual experiences. These experiences include a feeling of using their eyes in a peculiar manner in order to see properly, for example, eyes feel 'out on stalks'[5]. Patients who talk about having to 'use their eyes' in some strange way give a significant pointer to neurosis*.

Examination discloses for the most part negligible or quite minor optical errors. If glasses are proposed, most of these patients respond favourably either through anticipation of total relief or as a screen behind which they may hide. Other people can be observed through the apertures yet the patient feels cocooned from the cut and thrust of the real world. If prescribed, the symptoms usually disappear for a time, but as the placebo effect wanes they recur. A certain indicator of uncovered aetiology is the recurrence of the original symptoms after a period of relief with a new prescription.

Schizophrenic patients or those under the effects of hallucinogens present gross disorders of visual perception including palinopsia or delayed perception. The patient reports, for example, attempting to walk out of a door but finds instead a solid wall[6], indicating a transference of a previously true visual perception to a later, changed state. Shifts in spatial perception take place in that the patient feels removed from normal visual space, the environment fragments or becomes totally unreal[5]. The overriding neurological or psychotic state must receive attention.

Visual unease in decreased contrast sensitivity

Arden[7] reports conditions akin to visual unease in patients suffering from loss of contrast sensitivity, as in demyelinating disease. The patients are conscious of some difficulty with vision yet their account of this difficulty is vague. Visual acuity is normally measured by standard methods such as Snellen-type letters. Decreased contrast sensitivity is an early indicator to a range of diseases including certain forms of glaucoma, diabetes and multiple sclerosis, and the assessment of contrast sensitivity by the use of gratings is set to become a valuable clinical test method for the consulting room, especially so for patients who present visual problems but who are unable to give positive subjective guides to those problems.

References

1. PERKINS, G.D. and ROSE, F.C. (1976). 'Uhthoff's syndrome'. *Br. J. Ophthal.*, **60**, 60
2 REGAN, D., MURRAY, T.J. and SILVER, R. (1977). 'Effect of body temperature on visual evoked potential delay and visual perception in multiple sclerosis.' *J. Neurol. Neurosurg. Psychiat.*, **40**, 1083
3 CHAMBERLAIN, W. (1971). 'Restriction in upward gaze with advancing age.' *Am. J. Ophthal.*, **1** (Pt. 2), 341–346
4 DREWS, R.C. (1967). 'Organic versus functional ocular problems.' *Int. ophthal Clin.*, **7**, 665–696
5 HEATON, J.M. (1968). *The Eye: Phenomenology and Psychology of Function and Disorder*, p. 266. London: Tavistock and Lippincott
6 Personal patient report
7 ARDEN, G.B. (1978). 'Visual loss in patients with normal visual acuity.' Doyne Memorial Lecture. *Trans. ophthal. Soc. U.K.*, **98**, 219–231
8 NEMA, H.V. (1973). *Ophthalmic Syndromes*, p. 311. London: Butterworths
9 NEMA, H.V. (1973). *Loc. cit.*, p. 202

---

*This must be distinguished from peculiar or strange sensations which could be an indicator to early cranial tumour.

Chapter 7

Colour vision problems

'There's nothing wrong with my colour vision . . . it's only those pictures of coloured dots which get me confused'

Colour vision problems presented by patients are considered under two headings: congenital colour vision deficiencies; and colour vision deficiences manifested during life.

Congenital colour vision deficiencies

Patients who have one of the common sex-linked varieties of congenital colour vision anomaly (*Table 7.1*) rarely present symptoms. They often voice vocational problems but it is unusual for such a patient to make an unprompted observation about difficulty in distinguishing colours. An emphatic complaint from a patient relating to colour vision other than vocational problems should arouse suspicion of some acquired abnormality. A patient will sometimes comment: 'I know that I am colour blind' but not project their deficiency as presenting symptoms. They will agree, when asked, that some colours are confused, but usually approach these matters with good

TABLE 7.1. Approximate Frequencies (%) of Congenital-type Colour Vision Deficiencies (Caucasian)

| | Protan-type | | Deutan-type | | |
	—Anopia	—Anomaly	—Anopia	—Anomaly	Total
Males	1	1	1	4.5	7.5
Females	0.025	0.025	0.025	0.425	0.5

humour and without tension. If patients do have a problem arising from a congenital-type colour defect then it is likely to take the form of seeking an opinion on the state of colour vision for occupational purposes, such as entering a government service or industrial organization where some requirement regarding normality of colour vision has to be satisfied. These patients often admit to past indications of abnormality, for example, evidence from previous Ishihara test results seen at school or college, from an earlier eye examination or from incidents in which they have been found to confuse colours in their daily life.

Nevertheless, patients may reach quite a late age — 18 or 20 years is quite common — and yet be unaware of any anomaly[1]. This may not always be truthful reporting but a denial based on a previous psychologically disturbing experience. Minor deficiencies

61

pass unnoticed, either because the patient has learnt unknowingly to discriminate colours by apparent brightness difference or the defect is so slight that is poses no problems except under test conditions. Even if patients are aware of confusing colours some hesitate to disclose this, particularly if the patient is a young male having to cope with others of the same age. Occasionally, this leads to hypersensitivity, anxiety and aggression. Wearing contact lenses is something to boast about; making apparently stupid errors in colour discrimination is not. The congenitally colour defective person is still viewed with amusement by the lay public especially if they witness the colour confusions made in some practical situation.

Optometrists and others involved at this point in health care have an important role as educators and, whenever possible, should promote a better understanding of the problems encountered by the colour defective patient and encourage a shift in attitudes. Descriptions such as 'colour defective' or 'colour deficient', although used here and generally in the literature, should, preferably, be avoided in discussions with patients (*see* Chapter 3).

Colour confusions likely to be made by the congenitally colour defective patient

Real-life colour vision problems and clinical test confusions may not always fit neatly into the predicted patterns based on the psychophysical data of visual colorimetry, but it is useful to study these data.

The greater the degree of the defect, as in dichromatism, the more likely will problems have been noticed by the patient. If the protanope and deuteranope are examined using primary monochromatic spectral mixing stimuli in a spectroscopic-type instrument then there should be no hue discrimination in the red-green-yellow region. A spectral hue can be found which matches a defined white and at that point in the spectrum a 'neutral point' is said to occur. Both the spectral hue and the defined white will appear the same to the patient as the complementary colour, all three lying on a single confusion locus *(Figure 7.1)*. The spectral wavelength representing the neutral point will depend on the particular 'white' stimulus chosen, but is around 500 nm in deuteranopia (a greenish blue-green) and 495 nm in protanopia (a bluish blue-green). The complements of these neutral points are a purple and near-red respectively.

Why should these characteristics of the dichromat as determined in the vision laboratory not always be reflected into the presenting symptoms in the consulting room, in daily life, nor indeed always confirmed by conventional clinical methods of testing? The following reasons are the most important.

(1) Non-spectral colours are present in most clinical tests and in the environment. The confusion colours of the dichromat as predicated above are determined using spectral stimuli and these conditions are unlikely ever to be reproduced away from the vision science laboratory.

(2) The quality and intensity of illumination used in clinical testing will not usually conform to standard illuminants and the colour rendering of the sources used will be different.

(3) The density of macular pigmentation varies with the individual.

(4) Experience in judging colour by luminance differences can lead apparently to correct recognition of colours in practical situations.

(5) Contrast between a colour and its background.

(6) Spectral hues are fully saturated, unlike most everyday circumstances.

(7) Psychological embarrassment on the part of the patient.

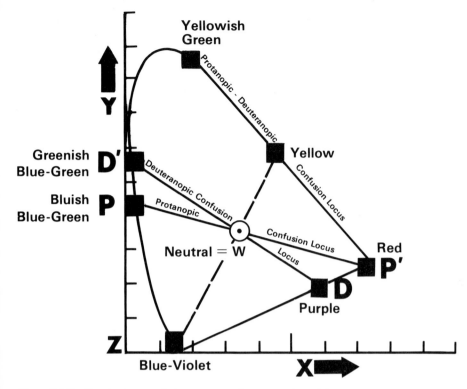

Figure 7.1. Predicted colour confusion symptoms in protanopia and deuteranopia from the data of visual colorimetry projected on to the C.I.E, XYZ chromaticity diagram. Deuteranopes match: (1) a greenish blue-green with grey and purple; (2) red-yellow and green. Protanopes match: (1) a bluish blue-green, grey and red; (2) red-yellow-green

Practical problems of the congenitally colour defective patient

Where there is a significant congenital colour defect, such as dichromatism or extreme anomalous trichromatism, then the patient will usually admit to confusion of some colours when questioned in the privacy of the consulting room and once confidence between the examiner and patient has been established. The following are some typical confusions reported by patients.

(1) Choosing clothes in apparently matching colours which, later, are shown not to match. In male patients this comment is often about neckties.

(2) Making faulty observations in scientific experiments at school. These include chemical analyses which have to be judged by colour change.

(3) Difficulty in discriminating colours in games such as snooker (especially reds and brown; brown and green).

(4) Problems in distinguishing between stained structures in histology (medical students especially) which appear to look the same. Haematoxylin/eosin stain proves to be difficult because of its pinks and purples.

(5) Using unusual colours in painting, for example, green grass is painted purple. This kind of error should not occur with single named paints, but it is a problem occasionally reported by patients when using paint mixtures.

The apparently colour deficient normal person

The normal person can appear to be colour defective under certain conditions. Some of these conditions are reproduced only in the vision laboratory, but others can be met in everyday life. Rarely, a normal patient may comment on some quirk of viewing conditions which has led to faulty observation.

The colour rendering of light sources

Street lighting from mercury or sodium vapour allows only poor or no colour discrimination. The subjective effect of 'white' light can be obtained, for example, by mixing blue and yellow lights only. Reds will be poorly discriminated in such a form of lighting.

Contrast effects

A transient anomalous trichromatism can be induced for a time by prolonged exposure to some colour. After long exposure to red light, then red/green anomaloscope matches of yellow will be abnormal if matching is attempted soon after removal of the red stimulus.

Foveal imagery

Vision becomes tritanopic if the retinal image is confined to the fovea.

Intensity of illumination

In very low illumination conditions reds become less easily distinguished. In very high illumination conditions desaturation of colours occurs.

Peripheral vision

Shifts of hue and saturation take place for small test objects viewed obliquely in the periphery as in perimetry. A saturated red progressively becomes orange, yellow then grey as the image moves from the fovea into the retinal periphery.

Brief flash

Colours are not perceived if the retinal illumination is brief, as from an electric spark.

Effect of distance

Small coloured areas undergo apparent changes of colour as they are moved from the observer into the distance — yellow appears white, blue tends towards black.

Stabilized retinal image conditions

Colours rapidly fade under stabilization of the retinal image.

Note:

The normal changes taking place in the crystalline lens with age gradually produce an acquired tritan-type defect.

Notes on the methods of examination for congenital defects

Full details of the methods used in the investigation of congenital colour vision deficiencies and the interpretation of the results of those tests are outside the scope of this book, but some general observations are presented on specific points.

The classification of a patient's defect into its trichromatic division (*Table 7.2*) is an interesting exercise but is unimportant in the consulting room. The main issue for the non-specialist practitioner is to determine whether a defect exists and, if so, its vocational significance.

One colour vision test may under-refer; another may over-refer so that a second, dissimilar test should always be used in any clinical examination. A third distinctly different method is useful in doubtful cases. Pseudo-isochromatic plates are most commonly used in practice, but no single set of plates will correctly classify the type and degree of all defects[2], indeed, some were designed solely from the observation of typical colour confusions made by defective individuals and were not intended to codify the findings in any but a very general way (for example, Ishihara plates).

TABLE 7.2. Classification of Defective Colour Vision—'Congenital-Type' Defects

	Trichromatism	
Deutan	*Anomalous trichromatism*	*Protan*
Simple deuteranomaly (DA)	Tritanomaly (TA)	Simple protanomaly (PA)
Extreme deuteranomaly (EDA)	Tetartanomaly (TTA)	Extreme protanomaly (EPA)
	Dichromatism	
Deuteranopia (D)	Tritanopia (T)	Protanopia (P)
	Tetartanopia (TT)	
	Monochromatism (achromatopsia)	
	Rod-cone type	
	Rod-type	

Notes:
(1) The abbreviations protan, deutan and tritan are used generally to include all variants in the appropriate category from minor anomalies through to dichromatism.
(2) This classification has evolved from the data of visual colorimetry to which other terms have been added from time to time, for example, tritanopia.

An acceptable consulting room technique combines pseudo-isochromatic plates and a lantern test for vocational examination. Those intending to specialize in the examination of colour vision should have some form of anomaloscope for the identification of the various forms of anomalous trichromatism.

A full battery of tests for the specialist might take the following form: (1) Ishihara and H.R.R. plates; (2) Edridge-Green, Giles-Archer or similar lantern test; (3) Nagel or Pickford-Nicholson anomaloscope; (4) Farnsworth 100 hue and 'D.15' tests; (5) standard illuminant.

There would be many variations on this theme in view of the wide range of clinical tests now available.

The patient should always be examined individually, unless a child with parents, and should not be subjected to mass screening if their errors in identifying charts or lights would thereby be on view to others.

Advising the patient who manifests a congenital-type colour vision anomaly

The first action should be to give an easily understood yet brief account of the reason for their problem. This might include reference to its congenital invariant and sex-linked nature and the probable effect on colour vision in causing colour confusions. The normality of vision in all other respects should be emphasized where this is the case. Some mention can be made of the conditions under which confusions are most likely to occur depending on the type and severity of the defect. In anomalous trichromatism, for instance, low brightness levels, poor weather, low colour saturations and small visual angles as well as fatigue — all can act to give misjudgements of colour. The safety implications should edge into the discussion without being introduced in such a way as to alarm the patient.

If the person is young, then either he or the parents should be advised of the occupational limitations imposed by defective colour vision and the need for school or college tutors to be aware of the problem. With the increasing use of automatic techniques, non-visual methods and computer assistance in industry, the range of occupations from which the colour defective patient is barred is decreasing. The aim should always to be prevent the young patient from becoming career-orientated at an early age with eventual exclusion, disappointment and wasted effort. Many occupations have their own official test procedures and it is the results of those examinations which determine acceptance or rejection. The practitioner can only act in an advisory capacity by giving an opinion unless authorized to carry out the official examination. It is advisable to keep up-to-date copies of the colour vision requirements governing the various occupations for which good colour vision is essential and these are best obtained locally in the individual country or state.

The fact that there is no known cure should be indicated to the patient although advice can be given, if requested, on minimizing the disadvantages of the defect. This advice must not be construed as recommendations to assist the candidate in attempting to pass some official test.

If the defect is not extreme then the advice offered can be along the following lines.

(1) The use of high illumination for better discrimination.

(2) Empirically prescribed absorption filters used successively may allow better discrimination of confused colours. As an example, red and green filters used successively have the following effect: a red coloured object appears to lose brightness through the green filter but not through the red one. A yellow object looks approximately equally bright through each filter whilst a green object becomes darker when viewed through the red filter. With the assistance of a normal observer the candidate can learn to recognize confused colours given a selection of tinted lenses. This form of assistance is useful for students of histology.

(3) The possibility of other types of coloured filter being useful, such as the 'X Chrom' lens.

(4) Using special markings on clothes which have confused colours.

(5) Avoiding the conditions under which colour discrimination is more difficult, for example, enlarge the visual angle; enhance the colour brightness.

(6) Take along a friend who has normal colour vision when choosing coloured articles in shops.

A somewhat delicate situation arises where the existence of a congenital colour vision defect could affect a patient's employment yet be unknown to the employer. Practitioners should be careful to hold discussions with the various bodies in industry before carrying out colour vision screening for research purposes, for statistical investigations or even just for interest. Great care must be taken in the use of the results of colour vision examinations or of records of discussions with patients as in all clinical work.

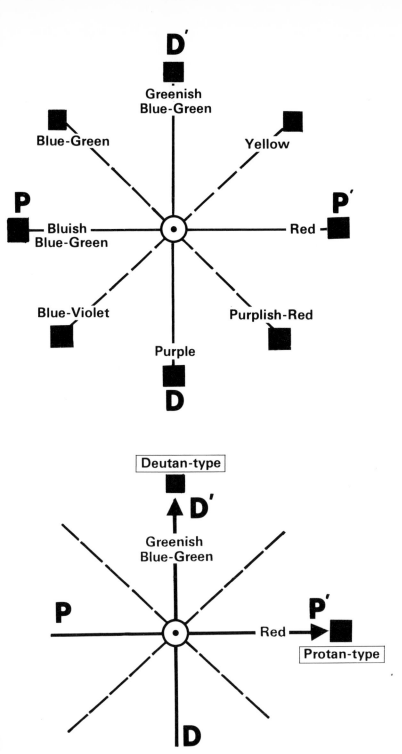

Figures 7.2 and *7.3*. Schematic representation of protan-deutan colour vision defects for clinical recording purposes. Axes PP′ and DD′ are taken as horizontal and vertical (*see Figures 7.1* and *7.4*)

Clinical recording of congenital colour vision defects

The abbreviations DA, EDA, D and PA, EPA, P (*see Table 7.2*) provide a method of recording which avoids lengthy descriptions such as 'extreme deuteranomaly'. They are restrictive in so much as the language of origin may not conform to the language of receipt of the information, thus the abbreviations may or may not be appropriate to the recipient. The congenital defects have well established visual characteristics and the specialist in colour vision examination will have categorized the patient by those characteristics.

A simple symbolic representation for the protan-deutan group is shown in *Figures 7.2, 7.3* and *7.4*, and can be used in clinical records. The method can be expanded to cover the acquired deficiencies, but as the characteristics, diagnostic significance and pathology are less clearly understood, the method has limitations for those conditions. A full description is given elsewhere[3].

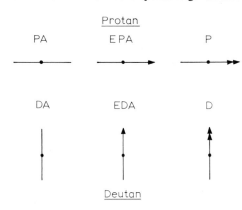

Figure 7.4. A method of clinical recording for the established degrees of severity of congenital protan-deutan colour vision defects

Colour vision deficiencies manifested during life ('acquired' colour defects)

If normal colour vision becomes abnormal during the life of an individual then an acquired colour vision defect is said to exist. The use of the word 'acquired' has been generally accepted in clinical investigations and research to include any deterioration of colour vision arising during life even if this originates from a genetically determined condition such as retinitis pigmentosa. Strictly, such disturbances in colour perception which have an underlying genetic base yet do not result in a measurable deterioration of colour vision until after birth should not be classed as 'acquired'. Nevertheless, the usage has become established.

Where an eye-related pathological condition acts to change the perception of colours, then the patient may present correlating problems in the history and symptom interview. If one eye only is affected, symptoms are less likely; the normal perception of the other eye overrides the abnormal perception in binocular superposition. Symptoms are most likely when the condition interferes with binocular macular function and take one or more of the following forms:

Confusion of colours in some practical situation

This may happen in the home, in leisure pursuits or at work. A patient, for example, who was later found to have a form of early progressive optic atrophy manifested the related change in colour vision when she began to paint designs on pottery in unusual colours during her work. Purple flowers and green leaves became interchanged and this deterioration in standard of work came to the attention of her supervisor[4].

Differences in colour values between the two eyes

This symptom should not be dismissed immediately as due to some oddity of lighting or to a similar accidental occurrence. Although the observation can occur in normal patients (*see* below) it is also a symptom arising from unilateral eye or related disease or from a condition more advanced on one side than the other. The colour changes noted result from the apparent desaturation of colours in the affected eye as in retrobulbar neuritis, or from the apparent changes in hue as from macular oedema where white objects may appear orange or some other colour (*see* page 73).

Normal patients sometimes complain of colour differences between their two eyes. There are many possible reasons for this observation but amongst the most common is differential adaptation arising on waking where one eye is light adapted, the other still moderately dark adapted from the effect of blankets or pillows. Selective adaptation of one retina also occurs from bright but oblique sources such as the sun or strong eccentrically placed artificial lights. If these normal appearances are to be discounted then the conditions under which the colour difference is noted must be fully explored and then correlated with other possible symptoms and signs.

Faulty colour naming

A patient whose colour vision changes during life possessed normal colour vision previously at some stage. The names of colours will have been learnt by the sensation aroused. If some other colour later arouses that same sensation then the original colour description attributed to that sensation may be used in describing that other colour. Colour naming tests such as lantern tests therefore have some marginal use in the examination for changes in colour vision arising early in eye diseases[5], but they have limitations and should always be used in conjunction with other methods of examination.

Coloured vision (chromatopsia)

Coloured vision is not a common symptom reported in the consulting room, but occasionally it precedes other changes in colour perception and may be one of the first indications of abnormality. There can be a complaint of coloured vision in photopic conditions or of colours being 'seen' when in darkness or with closed eyes[6]. The types of chromatopsia are dealt with on page 73.

Variations in colour vision

Transient changes in colour vision take place as the condition progresses, varies or recovers. Certain forms of toxic amblyopia show recovery when the toxin is reduced or ceased and if the condition is not too far advanced, colour vision and visual acuity slowly return to normal or near-normal.

Other distinguishing features of acquired colour vision deficiencies

A history of previously normal colour vision is, of course, significant. The ophthalmoscopic picture must be closely studied for signs of abnormal change. In early or moderately advanced stages of disease other correlating symptoms and signs are usually present. These include reduced visual acuity, visual field changes, abnormalities in dark adaptation or in the critical fusion frequency of flicker. The results of electrodiagnostic tests or fluorescein angiography may also be abnormal.

In the very early stages of some eye diseases, colour vision changes are claimed to be demonstrable before other symptoms or signs manifest themselves[7], but it is doubtful whether the practitioner in general practice will be able to give sufficient time to the detailed examination of colour vision required to show such very early changes.

The characteristics of the congenital varieties are well documented and placement into the traditional divisions and subdivisions is usually possible given a battery of tests including at least one using spectral stimuli. Acquired defects often give atypical results compared to the congenital varieties, and do not fit easily into the classical categories although at certain stages of a disease this may be possible.

Having regard to the complexity of the channels serving colour vision and with the intricate physiology not yet fully understood, then it is little wonder that the changes manifested in colour vision in diseased conditions show so wide a variation.

Related physiology

A section of the retina shows many cells but these typical sections do not show the meshwork of pathways available for intercommunication or for 'crosstalk' between those cells. It is now accepted that the input into the visual system which results in colour perception lies through three photopigments at the receptor or cone level of the retina. These first-stage signals are relayed and recoded within the retina via 'colour-coded' horizontal, bipolar and amacrine cells. This recoding results in opponent-type chromatic signals being then relayed into the optic nerve through colour-coded ganglion cells along with luminosity signals. The simple model (*Figure 7.5*) can give no precise indication of how that recoding takes place nor indeed of the inhibitory and excitatory gateways and mesh of communicating pathways which have evolved to make this processing possible.

Many authoritative works are now available dealing with the results of recent research in colour vision physiology and the physiology of vision (*see* Further reading). Only when this intimate physiology is fully understood will it be possible to predict with confidence the variations in vision and in colour vision to be expected from lesions affecting one or more parts of the retina or pathways. One condition in its early stages may attack the nuclei of certain forms of ganglion cell only; another may shift the balance of inhibitory impulses on those cells; yet another may selectively disrupt relays only in the inner nuclear layer. Each condition will have its unique stamp on the light perception process and will pass through its various stages to reach its full potential for damaging vision unless arrested or reversed spontaneously or by treatment.

Clinical examination

The clinical examination for defective colour vision will be dealt with only in brief. Details of examining techniques are not the primary purpose of this book; nevertheless, some comments which link these techniques with the symptoms reported by patients especially in the acquired disturbances are useful in analysing history and symptom data.

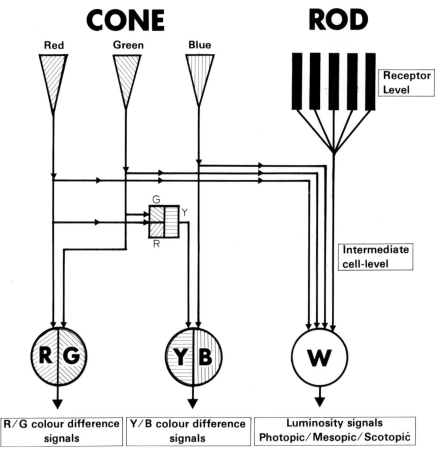

Figure 7.5. Trichromatic input — opponent output retinal model of colour and luminosity signalling

In many cases of acquired colour vision deficiency the test results do not conform to those expected for the typical congenital-type defects. Additionally, blue-yellow type changes are as commonly met as those of red-green and sometimes it is impossible to relate the changes to any of the typical results found in the congenital variations. Some conventional methods of examination used in vocational colour vision testing are unsuitable for the examination of suspected acquired anomalies if they do not allow for the investigation of blue-yellow, that is the tritan, series of colour vision change. The Ishihara series of pseudo-isochromatic plates have no charts specifically designed for that type of investigation.

There is a considerable and accumulating literature on the use of standard colour vision tests or their variants in a multitude of eye and related diseases. As a record of data corresponding to a certain condition then there is a well established clinical use but little further progress can be achieved in the understanding of the physiological basis of colour vision by using conventional clinical tests or their modifications in the examination of diseased eyes. If acquired colour vision deficiencies are to yield new information relevant to the physiology of the human colour vision process then progress is likely to come from methods using true spectral stimuli or from new methods designed around the use of such stimuli.

Tests such as the 100-hue test when used in the examination of acquired colour vision defects present information which is unique to that test[8]. Because of this test dependency the results of individual tests should never be treated in isolation from other basic and problem-oriented data for the patient. For this and other reasons a battery of tests is even more necessary for the examination of the patient to determine the presence of colour vision changes from disease than for vocational examination. The time taken to perform this battery of test methods will prelude their use as part of a normal eye examination. The minimum test procedures recommended for a full clinical examination would be Ishihara; H.R.R. or similar plates; lantern test for colour naming; Nagel or Pickford-Nicholson anomaloscope; Farnsworth 100 hue and D.15 tests; peripheral colour perimetry.

In the vision research laboratory, spectral hue discrimination and luminous efficiency functions are desirable data. Tests using coloured pigments such as pseudo-isochromatic plates should be used under standard illuminant conditions. For the colour vision examiner in practice then colour matching fluorescent or North Sky illuminants are satisfactory. Most forms of fluorescent lighting if not too 'warm' are acceptable alternatives.

Conditions which result in colour vision disturbances

An extensive literature exists dealing with the effect on colour perception of drugs, chemicals, diseases and other related conditions. The most important features only are reported here with the emphasis on possible presenting symptoms.

The Köllner rule

The perimetric rule attributed to Köllner (1912) gives a coarse guide to the changes in colour vision to be expected in conditions affecting the eye and optic pathways, thus: a red-green defect results from lesions of the optic nerve and optic pathways whereas a blue-yellow defect is associated with lesions of the retinal sensory epithelium, that is, the rod and cone layer.

This so-called rule should be applied with some caution. Marre, for example[9], considers that an isolated defect of the blue mechanism is usually the first manifestation of acquired deficiencies. In the early stages of disease there may be small losses of discrimination in various regions of the spectrum which will not fit any of the protan-deutan-tritan groupings as required by the rule. In the late stages of disease then conventional clinical colour vision tests are difficult to perform due to field loss or visual acuity changes and any results obtained will be quite anarchic. Dubois Poulsen[10] takes the view that the exceptions to the simple red-green/blue-yellow rule are so numerous that generalizations of that nature are of doubtful use.

Sometimes a patient is examined at a stage where the test results fit the characteristics of one of the congenital-type conditions as shown in the results, for example, of the Farnsworth-Munsell 100-hue test, such that a protan-deutan or tritan change can be distinguished. In other cases there is little similarity to congenital-type 100-hue results or there may appear to be an overlapping of two basic forms of congenital defect.

TABLE 7.3. Conditions in Which the 100-hue Test Results and Other Clinical Colour Vision Test Findings Correspond to the Tritan-Deutan-Protan Characteristics of Those Tests at Some Stage of the Development of the Named Conditions

Yellow-blue (tritan)	*Red-green (D = Deutan : P = Protan)*
Glaucoma	Optic atrophy in various forms (D)
Retinal detachment	Retrobulbar neuritis (D)
Retinitis pigmentosa	Chiasmal lesions (D)
Retinopathy in various forms	Juvenile macular degeneration (P)
Senile macular degeneration	Toxic amblyopia (D)
Papilloedema	Dominantly inherited juvenile optic atrophy (P)
Use of oral contraceptives	

With these reservations in mind, conditions in which acquired defects have been reported to mimic at some stage the results obtained in congenital deficiencies are as shown in *Table 7.3*.

Dependent symptoms

Colour vision dependent symptoms arising from disease or other disorders which affect colour perception may not be reported in terms which immediately identify the complaint as a colour problem. The patient may merely suggest that '. . . things seem to look brighter with this eye. . .' and visual acuity and other functions tested in routine eye examination may all appear to be quite normal.

The consulting room test chart may be described as 'off white' in macula oedema[11] or a yellow and violet annular appearance be observed when viewing a moderately illuminated white surface, such as a ceiling[14].

The following are other symptoms reported.

Faces seem duller with one eye than with the other (disseminated sclerosis with normal visual acuity).

Gold objects appear silver[12].

Mistaking a jar of pickles for red jam[13].

The patient's own appearance (in mirrors) or friends' complexions appear pale and ill-looking[12].

Painting in unusual colours[4].

Colours all appear 'muddy'.

Pruning green shoots in gardening which, through looking brownish, seem to be dying[14].

Where the changes are unilateral then the defect is noticed only when that eye happens to be used alone as when looking through a monocular viewing instrument such as a microscope, or when the 'good' eye is occluded accidentally.

Chromatopsia '. . . like looking through a pink mist . . .'

Chromatopsia, or coloured vision, is an abnormal perception of colour over the whole visual field as though the person were looking through a coloured filter. The various forms of coloured vision complained of by patients have been given names derived from classical origins. In order of general use these are as follows.

Name	Form of coloured vision
Erythropsia	Red
Xanthopsia	Yellow
Cyanopsia	Blue
Chloropsia	Green
Glaucopsia	Blue-grey
Ianthinopsia	Violet
Leucopsia	White

Coloured vision is not a common symptom reported by patients. One of the reasons for this lack of comment is progressive adaptation to the new visual conditions where the disease or abnormality is advancing only slowly. Chromatopsia arises in several ways as follows.

Selective absorption or scattering of light by the eye structures or in the prereceptor retina

Many drugs and eye disorders act on the prereceptor structures to give selective absorption of light. Any chemical or drug which has the action of colouring the transparent structures or the sclera alters the quality of light falling on the sensory receptors and, if the change takes place rapidly so that adaptation does not occur, then chromatopsia may be complained of. Mepacrin, for example, one of the older anti-malarial drugs used during World War II was occasionally a cause of transient xanthopsia from the yellowish discoloration of tissues. The topical application of fluorescein, as in contact lens practice, may also lead to a yellowing of the environment as a very temporary effect; indeed, any dye used topically in eye examination or treatment can act as a transient absorption filter.

Some other conditions which cause selective absorption are as follows.

Bile disorders (xanthopsia or ianthinopsia)   The sclera and cornea become pigmented and the yellowish deposits cause vision to be comparable to the world seen through a yellow filter. At times, vision may change to the complementary colour, that is, blue-violet. With a slow discoloration patients adapt to the new visual conditions and will not report symptoms of chromatopsia. Some degree of tritanomaly should be evident on examination with methods designed to demonstrate that condition.

Vitreous haemorrhage (erythropsia)   Objects in the environment appear as though seen through a red haze. When the haemorrhage is massive then vision is almost entirely lost, at least for a time, until absorption begins to take place. In a young person this is usually quite rapid.

Diffuse corneal or vitreous opacities (cyanopsia)   Dust-like particles in the cornea or in the vitreous humour scatter blue light preferentially akin to atmospheric scattering which produces the blue effect of the sky. The retina becomes suffused with blue light and, uncommonly, a patient may complain about the unnatural appearance of the environment.

Post-operative aphakia (transient erythropsia, cyanopsia, chloropsia, xanthopsia)   Reports of coloured vision following cataract surgery are numerous and cover most of the varieties of chromatopsia with erythropsia and cyanopsia predominating.

The ageing crystalline lens undergoes pigmentary changes as well as other chemical change and sclerosis. The yellowish pigment increasingly present with age reduces the retinal illumination compared to youth and shifts the spectral distribution of the light incident on the sensory retinal elements. A tritanomalous condition can sometimes be demonstrated attributable, at least in part, to the increasing lack of short wavelengths reaching the retina. This slow shift with age is unlikely to lead to a complaint of xanthopsia due to progressive adaptation. With the sudden removal of the crystalline lens, short wavelengths reach the retina in greater quantities than previously. The reversion to a more normal retinal spectral distribution gives rise to symptoms including coloured vision. The simple deduction that vision should become 'bluer' is not always borne out in the patient's complaint. Blue, red, green or yellow vision have all been reported as have other changes in colour vision and therefore prior conclusions on the eventual effect in an individual patient of removal of the crystalline lens can only be speculative.

Action of toxins, disease, trauma or excess radiation at various levels of the visual pathway

In diseased conditions, chromatopsia, if reported at all, is a likely forerunner of some deterioration in colour vision measurable by conventional clinical methods of examination, unless the disorder is arrested or reversed.

The conditions in which chromatopsia has been noted are varied and numerous. Lists of drugs, chemicals, toxins and diseased states in which coloured vision of some form has occurred can be found in other publications (*see* Further reading). General observations are given here together with typical examples from clinical practice.

Action on retinal receptors or on other cells of the retina   Over-exposure to visible radiation or to ultraviolet light has resulted in erythropsia, chloropsia and 'leucopsia' in which the environment appears bathed in white mist. Desaturation of colours occurs naturally after long exposure to bright light, even through closed lids, as in sunbathing. This alteration in colour values is unlikely to be remarked upon by any but the neurotic patient. Where there has been exposure to intense visible or ultraviolet radiation then typical complaints arise, as in 'snow blindness'. Not only may this kind of exposure lead to phototraumatic keratoconjunctivitis, but to other symptoms such as erythropsia and permanent colour vision changes.

Retinal and choroidal disease may, rarely, precipitate red, blue, green or violet vision. Erythropsia occurs in retinitis pigmentosa in some patients.

Optic nerve and optic pathways   Various forms of optic atrophy in their early stages sometimes give rise to symptoms of coloured vision including erythropsia, cyanopsia and ianthinopsia. These have included syphilitic, Leber's, tabetic and other uncommon forms which the optometrist in general, as opposed to hospital, practice is unlikely to encounter more than a few times in a practice lifetime.

Visual cortex and central areas   Exaggerated colour experiences and coloured vision are common in the misuse of psychotomimetics such as LSD 25 and mescaline. Ethyl alcohol and cannabis and derivatives of opium are other causes of chromatopsia. Enhanced colour contrast effects have also been reported in cranial tumour and in hysteria.

Coloured vision in normal individuals

Forms of coloured vision occur normally and the practitioner must be on guard against assuming that all such complaints arise from some abnormality of, or affecting, the visual system, or from the adverse effects of medication.

No experienced examiner would make such an assumption if a patient merely reports seeing coloured fringes around test chart letters or astigmatic fan lines at some stage of a subjective eye examination, for this is a common enough observation and the effect disappears once an existing ametropia has been fully corrected. However, some other comments of normal patients regarding coloured vision are worthy of mention.

Shadows seen in near-monochromatic light appear tinged with the complementary colour, a normal contrast phenomenon. Red night lights or red photographic lights give green shadows. Strong oblique illumination through the sclera from ground-located floodlights gives a transient erythropsia to those passing by. (Often, this kind of illumination of the eye also gives a magnificent entoptic demonstration of the retinal vessels seen against a red field.) Direct sunlight passing through the sclera causes the black print of reading matter suddenly to turn 'blood' red and this phenomenon may alarm a susceptible patient and be reported in the history interview.

Absorption lenses which do not absorb neutrally across the visible spectrum, will at first give coloured vision but this appearance rapidly disappears with adaptation. When the lenses are removed, complementary hues lighten up the visual field for a time. Patients realize the lens dependence of the effect and, because they do not understand the reasons for it, may remark on such manifestation during discussion of the history of wearing tinted lenses.

References

1 BALL, G.V. and BOLTON, R.H. (1957–67). Unpublished information. University of Birmingham (England), Freshmen Screening
2 PAULSON, H.M. (1974). 'Congenital colour deficiencies.' *Mod. prob. Ophthal.,* Colour vision deficiencies, II. **13**, 363–368
3 BALL, G.V. (1974). 'Terminology of colour deficiency.' *Mod. prob. Ophthal.,* Colour vision deficiencies, II. **13**, 354–362
4 BALL, G.V. (1974). 'Developments in the investigation and aetiology of colour deficiency.' *J. Soc. occup. Med.,* **24**, 54–58
5 WRIGHT, W.D. (1972). 'A survey of methods used in examining macular colour vision.' *Mod. prob. Ophthal.,* Acquired colour vision deficiencies. **11**, 2–11
6 MARRÉ, M. (1973). *The Investigation of Acquired Colour Vision Deficiencies, Colour '73* pp. 99–135. London: Hilger
7 LAKOWSKI, R. (1968). 'The Farnsworth–Munsell 100-hue test.' *Ophthal. Optician,* **8**, 862
8 ASPINALL, P.A. (1974). 'Some methodological problems in testing visual function.' *Mod. prob. Ophthal.,* Colour vision deficiencies. **13**, 2–7
9 MARRÉ, M. (1974). 'Colour vision and the "pill".' *Mod. prob. Ophthal.,* Colour vision deficiencies, II. **13**, 345–348
10 DUBOIS POULSEN, A. (1972). 'Acquired dyschromatopsias.' *Mod. prob. Ophthal.,* Acquired colour vision deficiencies. **11**, 84–93
11 SCHMIDT, I. (1973). 'On acquired colour deficiencies.' *Optom. Wkly,* **64**, (2), 34–38
12 HARRINGTON, D.O. (1964). *The Visual Fields,* pp. 212–213. St. Louis: Mosby
13 HEATON, J.M. (1968). *The Eye, Phenomenology and Psychology of Function and Disorder,* pp. 170–171. Philadelphia: Lippincott. London: Tavistock Publications
14 Clinical personal report

Further reading

BOYNTON, R.M. (1979). *Human Colour Vision.* New York: Holt, Rhinehart & Winston

CORNSWEET, T.N. (1970). *Visual Perception.* New York: Academic Press

LYLE, W.M. (1974). *Drugs and Disease Conditions which may Affect Colour Vision,* parts I & II. Ontario: University of Waterloo

PADGHAM, C.A. and SAUNDERS, J.E. (1975). *The Perception of Light and Colour.* London: Bell

POKORNY, J. (1979). *Congenital and Acquired Colour Vision Defects.* New York: Grune and Stratton.

WRIGHT, W.D. (1969). *The Measurement of Colour,* 4th ed. London: Hilger

Chapter 8

Headache as a presenting symptom

'. . . as though I'm wearing a concrete hat which is being pressed down tighter and tighter.'

Headache is one of a number of common problems where, in the absence of symptoms or signs suggesting otherwise, the consideration and elimination of ametropia and binocular vision anomalies is an essential early step in the event leading to ultimate diagnosis.

Generalized or localized ache or pain in the head is an everyday problem presented to the practitioner and its causes are numerous and often obscure. It can occur through some forms of refractive error or binocular vision problem but more commonly from over-indulgence in the so-called pleasures of life. The explanation may be as commonplace as mild anxiety or constipation, but it may be as potentially serious as leaking from an intracranial aneurysm.

The headache symptom presents a challenge for all those involved in primary health care. The integrated data obtained during eye examination sometimes holds the key to identification of the cause, and this being so and the headache symptom being frequently the main symptom in eye examination[1], then it is deserving of special attention.

Causes of head pain

The intricate physiological and neurological basis for headache and the anatomical pathways leading to localization is not a purpose of this book, but is covered in depth in texts devoted exclusively to head pain (*see* Further reading).

Headaches are likely to result where there is muscular tension or where dilatation, inflammation, pressure or traction affects parts of the intracranial vascular system. They are also much dependent on the life-style, personality and psychological state of the individual.

Some pathological states give severe headache with such other signs that the optometrist in general practice rarely becomes involved and, even then, only as intermediary to assist by emergency measures whilst medical attention is being arranged. An extreme example would be the intense occipital headache with partial or total loss of consciousness in subarachnoid haemorrhage.

Other headaches are less indicative of a pathological origin and duplicate those arising in many other bodily states, including ametropic conditions. The early stages of cranial tumour may involve the headache symptom and any practice having a random-based patient catchment will at some time have such a patient attend the practice — it may be the next patient on the appointment register.

The responsibility seems awesome, but just as the possibility must be faced it must not be allowed to precipitate a neurotic fixation on conditions of low probability. If there are no guiding symptoms or suspicious signs, if the headache has a relationship with vision/eye related activity and a functional eye disorder exists, then the highest probability is that the symptoms are associated with that disorder, or are of psychogenic origin. An opinion has to be formed based on the data collected and the observations made during the initial and any subsequent examination as to whether the information upholds a reasonable suspicion of some other abnormality even in the presence of an optically correctable eye disorder. In very early cranial tumour, for example, commencing optic disc congestion may be demonstrated or binocular co-ordination could be marginally affected. There may be evidence pointing to minor visual field disturbances in addition to headaches or there could be a report of unusual sensations or feelings. Notwithstanding the presence of significant ametropia a patient showing those signs or problems would be sent for further investigations.

'Characteristic' headaches

Tables have been produced from time to time setting out the probable aetiological origin of headache in terms of certain limited characteristics such as quality, intensity and location. The term *ocular headache* is often used. Tentative diagnoses based on the highly subjective judgement of quality and intensity, and on the more certain but still subjective opinion of location must be handled with extreme caution.

The main symptom of headache more than any other demands the integration of *all* data. Observations collected during eye examination and interview must then be related to each individual patient.

The quality characteristic most likely to be helpful in the final assessment is the judgement by the patients of pulsating sensations in their headache experiences. This kind of headache points towards a vascular origin but it must be remembered that the manner in which the practitioner presents questions influences the patient's answer, as does the patient's memory, so that an eye-related cause could never be ruled out on those grounds alone.

With these important observations in mind, the headache of refractive error and binocular vision disorder usually arises from anomalies of accommodation and convergence, such as early presbyopia, rarely with myopia, but often with uncorrected hypermetropia and binocular vision abnormalities, as in heterophoria. Most frequently it is described as a 'dull' ache; an ache 'behind the eyes' or around the brows; rarely at the vertex, but possibly occipital or temporal; a steady ache, arising near the end of the day but which may linger until the next morning. It must again be emphasized that no form of headache is specific to eye disorders.

The quality and intensity of headaches

In attempting to investigate the kind of feeling aroused in a patient by a headache the examiner impinges directly into the fundamental psychological area of sensory experience with all the inherent overtones of subjectivity and validity of methods of examination.

If the elementary pain sensation of all headaches resulting from a certain degree of uncorrected hypermetropia were identical, measured on some hypothetical objective scale, our experience of the reaction of individuals to that degree of uncorrected hypermetropia is one of continuing variety. One patient copes readily; another is prostrated.

A patient's inner experience of pain cannot be predicted or examined directly. It has to be deduced and assessed from observations which are assumed to indicate that experience. If patients are asked to find words or expressions to fit their past awareness of some unpleasant sensation the ability to do so will depend on: (1) the personality of the individual; (2) memory and recall of that experience; and (3) the possession of an adequate vocabularly from which to retrieve apt descriptions to represent that experience. (1) and (3) are connected insomuch as vocabulary is one indicator of intelligence.

Direct problem-oriented questions and their answers are of minor value except as a means of establishing rapport, as will be seen from the following.

> Q. *'How bad are your headaches?'*   A. *'They are very bad.'*
> Q. *'What do they feel like?'*   A. *'They are terribly painful.'*

A succinct unprompted account from patients regarding their headaches indicates little more than a high level of mental ability, rather than providing sound diagnostic clues. If the examiner wishes to probe the kind of feeling aroused, then a guiding framework must be provided within which the patient is offered the choice of alternatives which are as clearly different as possible.

It must be emphasized, however, that in this area, more than any other, the practitioner must be guarded in the weight to be put on these observations. Unpleasant experiences are more likely to be erased from memory than pleasant ones and the patient's recall of those experiences may suffer from unintended distortion or faulty elaboration. The patient's remembrances reflect personality and are influenced by the psychological state at the time of examination.

The semantic differential and the headache symptom

'I get a dull ache in my head.' In this typical description of a headache, the patient has unwittingly introduced one term from a qualitatively and grossly different couplet to express his feelings. 'Dull' and 'sharp' can be conceived as lying at the extremes of a particular rating scale and are termed a bipolar adjectival pair in behavioural research[2].

Dull ◄— Neither —► Sharp

'Is it a dull ache or a sharp ache?' is the type of question the examiner should pose to the patient. A guarded or equivocal response suggests that the particular couplet chosen does not seem relevant to that patient in assessing his feeling. The patient can either be presented with a forced choice of the simple dichotomy or the 'neither' possibility may be interjected.

Note:
A stepped rating scale can be conceived as lying between the extremes representing relative dullness or relative sharpness. The application of such stepped scales (usually seven point) is useful in behavioural research but less so in the context of the

optometric examination. The validity of the semantic differential for the assessment of feelings is also subject to some reservations.

It is not possible to recommend pairings suitable for each individual patient except to observe that the more extreme the acceptable pairings the more likely is the patient to be neurotic in temperament. For example, to the majority of people judging a headache in terms of 'bass' or 'soprano' seems ludicrous, yet the author knew one patient who insisted that her headaches were soprano, and thereby added a further indicator to the tentative diagnosis of psychoneurosis.

Two common headache-types (Patients 1 and 2) with grossly different characteristics are illustrated in *Table 8.1*. There is an infinite variety with apparent intensity of symptoms lying between and extending outwards from these two examples.

TABLE 8.1. Headache in Two Common Types with different Characteristics

	Patient 1 *(student aged 22 years)*	*Patient 2* *(clerical worker aged 22 years)*
Quality	Dull, steady, shallow	Dull, deep, throbbing
Intensity rating	Mild	Severe
Location	Brow, unilateral	Frontal, unilateral
Origin and onset	1 year ago	5 years ago; develop over 10–20 minutes
Association	With work for degree studies	
Periodicity	Frequent when, or after, studying	Frequent at any time
Duration	1–2 hours	Several hours
Prevention, intensification, relief	Less frequent in vacations	No prevention or relief found; alcohol seems to intensify
Effect on activities	Irritates, but work can continue	Work has to cease

Aetiological probabilities (where no other guiding symptoms or signs exist).
Patient 1
If clinical emmetropia is found and binocular vision is normal then the highest probability is of anxiety in the student-examination-studying context. Uncorrected hypermetropia, anisometropia, oblique astigmatism, near esophoria or negative physiological exophoria are other common causes.

Patient 2
Migraine is a prime condition for consideration. In older patients a hypertensive condition would also rank high as a causative factor.

The clinician in the consulting room office is not practising in the research environment of a psychological or behavioural studies laboratory but will find it useful to adapt techniques from these skills in phrasing problem-oriented questions to patients.

Opposing adjectival pairs are presented to the patient to give a coarse, but rapid judgement on quality and intensity of feeling.

Qualitative or evaluative pairings[2]

Dull . . . Sharp
Deep . . . Shallow (superficial)
Steady . . . Pulsating (throbbing, stabbing)

Intensity or potency pairings[2]

Mild . . . Severe
Weak . . . Strong

Most patients accept the above pairings and make a distinct choice, but some do not. Not all patients react to the same adjectival extremes; indeed, some seem quite irrelevant. Weak . . . Strong has the lowest acceptance of the above pairs in the context of a headache. Others are even less so, yet occasionally a patient accepts a rather unlikely couplet such as:

Heavy . . . Light   Rough . . . Smooth
Loud . . . Soft   Dark . . . Bright

but these are not recommended for general use.

Questioning the patient

Some forms of headache are more commonly described by patients than others in optometric practice. If the cause is not immediately obvious, information on the characteristics of a patient's headache has some use to set alongside the other data at the decision-making stage, *but it should never be considered in isolation.*

It has been emphasized previously that no form of headache is specific to eye-related problems either in general or in particular. Functional eye disorders may or may not cause headaches. Headaches which seem typical of such disorders may have a quite different cause. What is most important is that they should not be considered independently from the patient as an individual. The characteristics of the headache symptom most useful in considering their possible relationship to eyes are as follows.

Direct association with specific eye or vision-related activity

Headaches arising gradually during close work may be the result of accommodative stress, as in early presbyopia, uncorrected hypermetropia, convergence insufficiency, minor degrees of astigmatism or anisometropia. Headaches reported to occur immediately after commencing such close work are more likely to be due to psychoneurosis.

Onset, indicating association with specific eye/vision activity

Headaches occurring late in the day are often the result of close work carried out earlier in that day. They can occur in individuals who need no optical correction at all

TABLE 8.2. Headache — Some Aetiological Probabilities

Relatively common in general optometric practice	Relatively uncommon or rare in general optometric practice
Stress, muscular tension, anxiety, depression, overwork, insomnia	Chronic angle closure glaucoma
Over-indulgence, addiction (for example alcohol)	Retrobulbar neuritis
Fatigue, constipation	Raised intracranial pressure, brain abscess, tumour
Uncorrected or poorly corrected refractive errors	Ocular inflammations
Accommodation anomalies, heterophoria and other binocular vision anomalies	Fever, inflammation of cranial arteries
Undue physical activity	Subarachnoid bleeding
Migraine and its variants	Intracranial aneurysms
Adverse effects of drugs, toxins, exogenous, endogenous	Otitis
Vascular hypertension	Severe trauma
Minor trauma	Encephalitis
Foci of infection, oral, nasal sinuses	Deficiency diseases

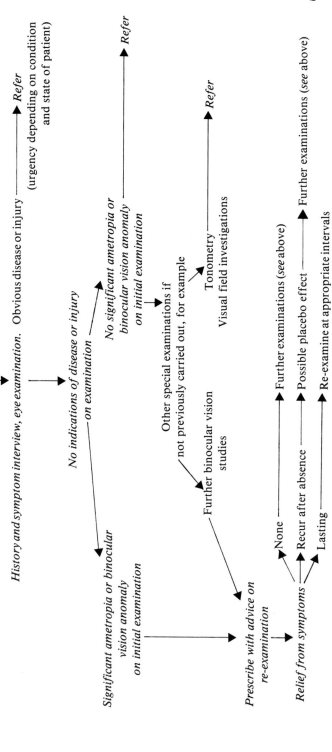

Figure 8.1. Optometric action flow diagram for patients presenting the symptom of headache

due to faulty reading posture, poor illumination, or in students, for example, who are anxious about poor performance in their academic work.

Prevention/relief

Relief obtained by refraining from close work occurring at weekends or during vacations points to a refractive/binocular vision/psychoneurotic disorder associated with work problems. A headache action flow diagram for optometrists is given (*Figure 8.1*) and some other causes of headache are ranked in *Table 8.2*.

Clinical characteristics of the headache symptom — Question schedule

Characteristics	*Suggested problem-oriented colloquial questions*
Quality Adjectival differentials such as: steady . . . pulsating; sharp . . . dull; deep . . . shallow	*See* previous paragraphs
Intensity Adjectival differentials such as severe . . . mild	*See* previous paragraphs
Location (site) in terms of skull reference Generalized, localized, frontal, brow, around eyes, temporal, unilateral, bilateral	'Can you point to the part of your head where you feel your headaches?' 'Are they always in the same place or not?'
Origin and onset Days, weeks, months (ago), sudden, gradual, on waking, end of day, nocturnal	'When did you first notice your headaches?' 'Do you get them at any particular time of day or night?' 'Do they come on suddenly or gradually?'
Association Reading, travel, television, sport, weather, work, sewing, theatre, stress, movement, posture	'Do they seem related to any activity?' (Examples may be given)
Periodicity Frequent, infrequent, occasional, regular, irregular, daily	'How often do you get them?'
Duration Transient, persistent, short, prolonged (minutes, hours, days)	'How long do your headaches last?'
Prevention: intensification: relief Refraining from activity, medication, rest, sleep, holidays, closing one or both eyes, head posture	'Have you found any way of preventing your headaches occurring or of relieving them?' 'Do you find anything makes them worse?'
Effect on activity Cessation, impairment, annoyance (maximal, minimal, nil)	'Some people have to stop work, activity or reading when they have a headache; others find they can carry on — how do you manage?'

Recording the details of the headache symptom

Abbreviations are sometimes recommended for quickly and accurately recording the patient's account of the headache symptom. Their use is a matter for individual preference. Personal shorthands are difficult for 'locum tenens' practitioners to interpret unless the abbreviations are universally recognized or an exact translation is kept in a prominent place. Unless the shorthand is used very frequently even the initiating examiner can be mystified when records are consulted years later.

For those who prefer some type of shorthand, the following abbreviations are in fairly general use.

Bilat.	= Bilateral		Fr.	= Frequent
Br.	= Brow		Grad.	= Gradual
Fron.	= Frontal		Infr.	= Infrequent
Occ.	= Occipital		Irreg.	= Irregular
Temp.	= Temporal		Occas.	= Occasional
Unilat.	= Unilateral		Pers.	= Persistent
V. or Vert.	= Vertex (Vertical)		Reg.	= Regular
			Rdg.	= Reading
			Trans.	= Transient

D.	= Dull			
Dp.	= Deep			
Gen.	= Generalized			
Loc.	= Localized		am.	= Morning
Mld.	= Mild		ev.	= Evening
Puls.	= Pulsating		h.	= Hours
Sev.	= Severe		m.	= Minutes
Sh.	= Shallow		Noct.	= Night
Shp.	= Sharp		pm.	= Afternoon

References

1 PICKWELL, L.D. (1960). 'The anatomy of headache.' *Br. J. physiol. Optics,* **17,** 151–160
2 OSGOOD, C., SUCI, G. and TANNENBAUM, P. (1957). *The Measurement of Meaning.* Illinois: University of Illinois Press

Further reading

HUBER, A. (1971). *Eye Symptoms in Brain Tumors,* 2nd ed. St. Louis: Mosby
WOLFF, H.G. (revised by DALESSIO, D.J.) (1980). *Wolff's Headache and Other Head Pains,* 4th ed. Oxford: Oxford University Press

Chapter 9

Patients' problems associated with mesopic and scotopic vision

'I don't seem to see very well in the dark now.'

Few patients present themselves in the consulting room office with true night blindness, yet that term is commonly used for any form of defective vision at low levels of luminance.

Night blindness is not therefore an ideal clinical description and, if used at all, should be restricted to the small numbers of patients who have no scotopic-type adaptation. Alternatively, it should be qualified by *incomplete* or *partial* in cases where good night vision is deficient but not entirely lost. *Defective* night vision is a better clinical description. Sometimes the words nyctalopia or hemeralopia are used to describe the absence of rod function but the former is correct on etymological grounds.

A typical comment from a patient heads this paragraph. 'I don't seem to see very well in the dark now.' What does the patient mean by 'don't seem to see very well?' Is the patient's vision affected generally in low illumination or in specific tasks only? What general levels of brightness are conveyed by the word *dark*? The inference of 'now' is that vision was better in the past. If so, over what period has it deteriorated? That seemingly simple statement by the patient must be examined on all those counts. Generally, patients who make such statements refer to vision out of doors at night in reasonable street lighting when involved in some visual task such as driving or as a pedestrian negotiating unfamiliar obstacles.

The luminance levels involved in those activities are not usually scotopic but fall into the mid-mesopic to upper mesopic range or into low photopic brightnesses. Scotopic luminances can simply be represented by vision on a clear moonless night with no artificial light sources whatsoever. Scotopic levels are rarely experienced by city dwellers. Night driving with headlights will bring most of the illuminated objects into the mesopic or low photopic values although luminances in night driving through country and city fall into all visual levels.

The examiner is nearly always concerned therefore with patients who have visual task problems as brightness levels approach and enter the mesopic range. Urban street environments at night give many problems for patients with cataract or other media anomalies.

Related physiology

When vision shifts from high to low luminance levels, characteristic and well-known changes take place (*Table 9.1*). In the literature of visual science the most celebrated of

TABLE 9.1. Characteristics of Normal Photopic and Scotopic Vision

Photopic	Scotopic
Visual acuity maximal at fovea	*Visual acuity and light sensitivity maximal off the fovea
Normal colour vision	*Achromatic vision
Normal visual field	*Central scotoma and possible enlargement of the blind spot
Average refractive state — clinical emmetropia (in young age-groups, slight hypermetropia)	*Average refractive state — relatively more myopic than photopic refraction
Clinical orthophoria at distance	Tendency to low luminance convergence
Normal accommodation for age	Tendency to low luminance presbyopia
Maximum luminous efficiency approximately 555 nm	Maximum luminous efficiency approximately 505 nm
Normal visible spectrum	Loss of luminous efficiency beyond approximately 680 nm

* These changes have the greatest clinical impact

hese changes is the shift in colour values (Purkinje phenomenon) but this is of minor clinical importance. The most noticeable subjective effect is the progressive sacrifice of other visual functions, such as high visual acuity and colour vision, to the detection of minute quantities of light. The retinal mosaic becomes coarse but highly powerful as a light gathering mechanism. Clinically, the change towards maximum visual acuity and light sensitivity away from the fovea: the development of a central scotoma and a myopic increase in refraction are the most significant for the normal patient.

The regeneration cycle of rhodopsin has long been acknowledged as having an important bearing on the increase in light sensitivity but the course of that regeneration could not by itself explain so massive a change in retinal sensitivity. Some form of correlating neural reorganization had to be involved. Work in lower animals shows that cones have a powerful inhibitory effect on rods in photopic conditions and that both rods and cones converge to single ganglion cells in the retina. The case for interaction between rods and cones as vision changes from photopic to scotopic levels is well founded but the exact physiological patterns have yet to be fully resolved. The anatomical routes for 'cross talk' amongst the receptors are numerous. It seems probable that some cones share with rods the same final pathways from certain types of ganglion cell and that it is the opening and closing of inhibitory gates on the retinal routes to those cells which allows signals either to flow or to be obstructed at various levels of luminance. During the intermediate stage of mesopic vision inhibition on rod summation is being removed so that the large numbers of rod receptors which converge on to bipolar cells are able to relay information through ganglion cells into the optic nerve channels. For fuller information on recent advances in the relevant physiology the reader is referred to the many journals on visual science and research in vision.

Causes of poor vision at low luminance levels

Reduction of pupil size with age

The decrease in the size of the pupil with increasing age has a profound effect for older patients and together with the need for presbyopic additions is the most common reason for reading problems in artificial lighting. The reduction in pupil aperture may be accompanied by a real elevation of the terminal light threshold in patients above the age of 70 years. There is also loss of transmission in the crystalline lens and vitreous humour.

All these factors combine to produce an increasing sense of difficulty in average room illumination for many patients in their advancing years — levels of illumination which would be quite adequate for younger individuals. Older patients feel that their vision is deteriorating and become anxious about possible blindness and cataract although they do not always ask direct questions, fearful that their suspicions will be confirmed. It is crucial, therefore, that the examiner reassures older patients if there appears to be no other problem than the need for increased illumination and spectacle reading additions (*see also* Glaucoma below). There is a responsibility on the practitioner to advise older patients on the types of and how best to arrange supplementary lighting, so that the problems associated with small pupils are minimized.

Ametropia

Patients' complaints about vision at low levels of luminance is not unusual as a symptom associated with refractive errors and this may be the simple answer to the problem. Myopes in need of a change in prescription complain of visual difficulty as daylight fades, especially in a visual task such as driving. Their need for additional negative power is compounded by the eye's normal shift to a relatively more myopic state with lowering luminance (night myopia; twilight myopia) and vision becomes noticeably worse.

The need for the correction of a refractive error or for the adjustment of an existing prescription is the most common explanation for mild complaints about twilight vision amongst patients who present themselves for eye examination. Refractive errors which the practitioner may feel diffident about correcting for photopic conditions assume a greater importance at mesopic levels. Small myopic errors which in youth are largely compensated by the small pupils of photopic vision may become intolerable to a few hypersensitive patients as the change from photopic into mesopic vision occurs.

Media changes

Irregularities in the optical media of the eye, particularly in the cornea and crystalline lens rank high in the list of conditions causing poor vision at dusk or at night. Early cortical cataract gives irregular refraction, scattering of light and reduces the illumination of the retinal image. In photopic vision, the contracted pupil nullifies much of the effect, but if the pupil has a normal dilatation there is a marked influence in mesopic conditions. Patients with early senile-type cortical cataract and other forms of lenticular opacity find difficulty in driving at night although their photopic acuity may be quite satisfactory for these tasks.

These media conditions are readily identified during normal eye examination. If adaptometry is carried out using a spot source, then, unless the media changes are considerable, the terminal dark adaptation threshold may not appear to be abnormal, but if visual acuity is determined under decreasing luminance, it will show a marked deterioration from normal values for that age-group for the level of mesopic luminance considered.

Glaucoma

Visual difficulty in reading under artificial lighting or in night driving always warrants some form of check for glaucomatous conditions unless the explanation for the problem is apparent. Elevated terminal thresholds have been reported to occur in the non-acute or sub-acute varieties such as chronic angle closure glaucoma[1,2]. Patients sometimes complain of problems in moving from one level of illumination to another, for example, when entering a dimly illuminated corridor from a well-lit room.

Whether dark adaptation is affected in an individual, and if so, the stage at which this occurs, cannot be stated precisely. The use of adaptometry in the examination for these types of suspected glaucoma must be considered quite peripheral to the more immediate methods of confirmation, such as tonometry, ophthalmoscopy and the examination of central and peripheral fields.

Retinitis pigmentosa and its variations*

Because of its poor prognosis for vision and the widespread publicity which has recently been given to retinitis pigmentosa, there is a tendency for the condition to receive undue emphasis in a teaching curriculum and the likelihood of retention of the information in the early stages of professional practice is high. The presenting symptom of poor night vision, therefore, is most likely to precipitate fears in the examiner's mind of this form of retinal dystrophy but in general practice it is rarely seen. Genetically determined retinal dystrophies are more common to hospital practice, but even there the incidence of affected patients is low. Arakawa *et al*[3] during 11 years in the Out-patients Department of the Kyushu Hospital in Japan reported only a 1.1 per cent incidence of retinitis pigmentosa. There are probably significant geographical variations, but the optometrist in general practice will see few such patients in a lifetime devoted to eye examinations unless there are special factors such as proximity to a hospital eye department.

The probability that any individual patient complaining of poor vision at night is suffering from retinitis pigmentosa is low. In patients who have the early stages of the disease the history and symptom discussion may disclose the familial link, but it is the increasing difficulty of vision at low luminance levels which first brings the condition to the patient's attention, unless it is atypical or there has been prior counselling, or objective monitoring. An added problem reported by patients is in changing from different levels of illumination[4].

Electrodiagnostic techniques, particularly EOG and ERG investigations have become established for the detection and examination of the condition in its early stages[5]. Typically it shows a recessive mode of inheritance, but occasionally there can be dominant heredity. The dominant form has a better prognosis for the retention of useful vision to a late stage although the effect on dark adaptation in all forms is severe. The reader is referred to any of the many standard works which fully review retinitis pigmentosa and its variations.

Assisting the patient who has retinitis pigmentosa

In the course of their work it is possible that optometrists will be questioned by patients who have read about, or know someone who has, retinitis pigmentosa. The

---

*The term 'retinitis pigmentosa' is in common use both in medical and lay circles. Alternative terms such as 'primary pigmentary retinal dystrophy' which more accurately reflect the nature of the disease, have not been widely supported.

most common questions are whether there is a successful form of treatment or cure or whether the patient can be asisted in any way. Here, the ability to communicate helpfully will prove invaluable.

A highly guarded response to the question of treatment is prudent until there is acceptable scientific evidence that the condition can be arrested by any particular mode of intervention, such as tissue therapy. Biomedical researches in genetic engineering may hold prospects for future prevention but these events have to be awaited and pose wider problems than those of retinitis pigmentosa.

On the question of assisting the patient who suffers from retinitis pigmentosa there can be marginally less pessimism, but determing whether the individual can be helped at all and, if so, the level of assistance possible, is time-consuming and needs skill and patience on the part of both examiner and patient. In the absence of techniques which are proved to arrest or reverse the condition the emphasis must always be on making the best possible use of remaining visual abilities. Lost vision cannot be regained. That message, if no other, *must* register firmly with the patient and with the immediate relatives if disillusionment, wasted time, irritation and criticism are to be avoided.

Having made those points then the methods of assistance fall into the following categories.

Correction of ametropia   It is simple to be so concerned with the underlying degenerative state that regular updating of the patient's optical prescription seems less urgent than discussions and palliative measures designed to help the patient psychologically. Significant ametropia must be meticulously corrected.

Absorption and other forms of lens   Complaints of photophobia are met in retinitis pigmentosa as also are the difficulties, mentioned previously, of moving from one level of illumination to a different, and lower one. Absorption lenses of various characteristics have been noted to assist some patients[11] although with this and with any form of attention the possibility of individual placebo effects cannot be discounted. Arbitrarily prescribed low-powered negative lenses are also said by some patients to be a help to them.

Field expanders   Patients who have severe field contraction with unimpaired central vision retain a high information channel capacity concentrated into a small percentage of the visual environment. Evidence supports the view that selected patients can benefit from the use of miniature optical systems which project a minified image of the environment on to the remaining functional area of the retina[6,7,8]. The devices can be offset into tinted spectacle lenses so that the patients can direct their attention to the minified image whenever an overall view of the environment is required, thus, at that moment 'enlarging' their field of vision. The tinted lens serves to alleviate any photophobia and disguises the presence of the miniature optical system (*Figure 9.1*).

The word *expander*, used in discussion with retinitis pigmentosa patients, might imply a real expansion of their field of vision, whereas the field is being optically minified to fit the remaining peri-foveal functional retinal area. The purpose of the system must be explained in advance so that there is no patient misinterpretation.

Both field expanders and image intensifiers (*see* below) are not available for trial by patients through the average practice and patients must be directed through recognized procedures to a centre which has the necessary staff and expertise to offer that form of service to the patient. The number of patients who can benefit from the

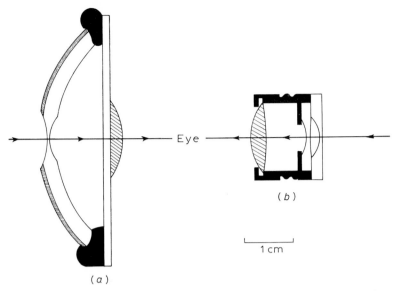

Figure 9.1. Two types of field expander (after Drasdo [8, 10]). (*a*) Surface-tinted lens incorporating an integral bioptic-type visual field expander. (*b*) A three-element optical system

use of field expanders is small. For those who can adapt, then the prospect of increased and easier mobility in strange environments is very welcome[9,10]. The number of researchers or practitioners who have the experience to advise on these special devices is very limited and the economics involved in the provision of such highly skilled time is a considerable limitation.

Image intensifiers   In the early stages of retinitis pigmentosa the lack of scotopic adaptation is a considerable handicap. Hand-held light intensifiers which shift mesopic and scotopic luminances to low photopic levels render objects visible which would otherwise be invisible[12,13]. The intensifier can be carried in the pocket or handbag ready for use when needed (*Figure 9.2*). Image intensifiers are not generally available and whether they would give assistance to the patient depends very much on the particular circumstances of each case.

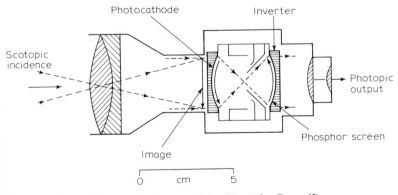

Figure 9.2. Image intensifier for defective night vision (after Berson[13])

Congenital (essential) nyctalopia

This familial abnormality is also uncommonly presented in optometric practice. The main symptom is always lack of good vision at low luminance levels. In the typically dominant form there are no other observable changes or symptoms other than those relating to mesopic and scotopic visual function. The modes of transmission are well established, there being dominant, recessive and sex-linked recessive varieties, the latter usually manifesting other symptoms or signs. Famous pedigrees exist such as that of the Nougaret family[14]. In the dominant form the patient is usually aware of the familial problem. Weale *et al.*[15] have demonstrated that rhodopsin concentration is normal in both recessive and dominant inheritance, suggesting that neural transmission is faulty. Because of the normality of photopic vision in the typical variety, image intensifiers could assist some patients who can adapt to their use (*see* above).

Dietary deficiency

In countries having a high standard of nutrition a primary diet-based disorder such as avitaminosis A is rare, although a secondary form of deficiency due to faulty absorption of the vitamin, as in liver malfunction, may eventually create ocular and visual problems for the patient.

In prolonged dietary lack of vitamin A, defective dark adaptation is reported to be one of the first symptoms along with dryness of the conjunctiva. Where the deficiency is experimentally produced, individual differences are found both in symptoms and in the normality or otherwise of dark adaptation at selected intervals of time. The susceptibility of the individual is therefore quite variable. Other vitamin (for example, B_2 and E) and dietary deficiencies are also thought to be associated with poor night vision although lack of vitamin A is the classic offender. The 'attacks' of night blindness reported over the years in orphanages, armies and in other civilian groupings were probably as much associated with hysteria as with true dietary problems.

Psychoneurosis

A disturbing experience at night, such as an automobile accident or a street attack can precipitate an hysterical reaction related to the conditions prevailing at that time. The patient may find it impossible to carry out normal activities at night, yet visual functions including adaptometric functions appear to be within normal limits or may show variable results. The history discussion assumes great importance in those cases. Electrophysiological investigations can demonstrate the normality of retinal function in scotopic conditions. Optokinetic nystagmus drum stripes are reported 'seen' later than the onset of the induced nystagmus as luminance is raised to a seeing from a non-seeing level. Hysterical nyctalopia is rarely encountered in general optometric practice.

Other conditions causing the symptom of poor vision at low luminance levels (*Table 9.2*)

Any abnormality affecting the functioning of the retina or the conducting pathways will have some effect on vision and this may involve mesopic and scotopic levels.

TABLE 9.2. Some Causes of the Symptom of Defective Night Vision

	Possible cause	*State of adaptometric terminal threshold, if measured*
Poor vision at low luminance levels	Uncorrected or poorly corrected refractive errors, especially myopia	Normal or near normal
	Age effect of small pupils	Normal or near normal
	Peripheral lens changes as in early senile-type cortical cataract	Probably within normal limits for the patient's age unless the condition is advanced
	Peripheral corneal irregularities	Probably within normal limits
	Some forms of glaucoma	Probably abnormal
	Retinitis pigmentosa and its variations	Highly abnormal as an early characteristic in both recessive and dominant inheritance
	Psychological problems including hysteria	Probably normal but may show fluctuations
	Congenital nyctalopia	No scotopic function
	Metabolic disorders including avitaminosis A Liver disease	Elevation of terminal threshold at some stage dependent on the individual
	Rare syndromes (for example, Uyemura's)	

Whether the effect is demonstrable subjectively will depend on the nature and degree of the condition and on the perceptive ability of the patient. Hypertensive retinopathy, macular degeneration, retinal oedema, retinal detachment, myotonic dystrophy, toxic conditions, diabetes — all have been reported at various times to give diminished dark adaptation.

Myopia has long been associated in the literature with defective dark adaptation but the evidence is indecisive. Where there are accompanying degenerative changes in the fundus, then vision will be affected in accordance with those changes, but unless the myopic error is large there is no firm evidence to link *uncomplicated* myopia with any marked effect on the terminal light threshold.

Notes on clinical examination

Adaptometry is of low priority in the investigation of patient's problems at low luminance levels. All the conventional basic data and much other problem-oriented data must be gathered before subjecting a patient to the time-consuming and fatiguing technique of subjective adaptometry. There must be the normal discussion of history and symptoms. If the cause remains obscure then the usual comprehensive eye examination must be carried out, including ophthalmoscopy and visual field investigations. From these routine methods the cause of the symptom can usually be identified unless it arises from a psychological disturbance. Only when all these investigations have been carried out with negative results should adaptometry be considered. Subjective adaptometry is not practicable in the restricted time of the conventional eye examination even if the practitioner has access to some form of adaptometer. Considerable experience in the technique is needed if consistent results are to be obtained and the spread of normal results is quite wide. Unless the course of dark adaptation and the terminal light threshold are markedly abnormal the results often lie within the normal limits for that patient's age-group.

In families with known pedigrees of congenital-type night blindness, investigation of the dark adaptation of affected members is quite academic and useful only for comprehensive case records or for demonstration purposes with the agreement of the patient.

It is useful to note that many early changes in the visual field can first be detected at mesopic luminance levels and a low luminance examination technique should be included in any thorough investigation.

References

1 ZUEGE, P. and DRANCE, S.M. (1967). 'Studies in the dark adaptation of discrete paracentral retinal areas in glaucomatous subjects.' *Am J. Ophthal.,* **64**, (i), 56–63
2 JAYLE, G.E. and OURGAUT, A.G. (1959). *Night Vision,* pp. 220–233. Springfield, Illinois: Thomas
3 ARAKAWA, T., NISHIMURA, M., INOMATA, H., NABESHIMA, T. and OSHIO, K. (1975). 'Pigmentary retinal dystrophy: statistical study of 572 cases.' *Folia ophthal. jap.,* **26**, 1036–1044
4 CURRIE, B. and DRASDO, N. (1977). 'A review of retinitis pigmentosa.' Internal Publication, Department of Ophthalmic Optics, University of Aston in Birmingham, England
5 GALLOWAY, N.R. (1975). *Ophthalmic Electrodiagnosis.* London: Saunders
6 HOLM, O.C. (1970). 'A simple method of widening restricted visual fields. *Archs Ophthal.,* **84**, 611–612
7 HOLM, O.C. (1975). 'Visual field widening in retinitis pigmentosa.' *Acta ophthal.,* Suppl. 125
8 DRASDO, N. (1976). 'Visual field expanders.' *Am. J. Optom. physiol. Optics,* **53**, 9, Pt. 1, 464–467
9 DRASDO, N. and MURRAY, I. (1978). 'A pilot study on the use of visual field expanders.' *Br. J. physiol. Optics,* **32**, 1, 22–29
10 BALL, G.V. and DRASDO, N. (1978). 'Optical and other aids for visually handicapped patients.' *Transactions of the International Symposium on Ophthalmological Optics, Tokyo,* **IV**, 1, 47–50
11 EVERSON, R.W. and SCHMIDT, I. (1976). 'Protective spectacles for retinitis pigmentosa.' *J. Am. optom. Ass.,* **47**, 738–744
12 SHAGEN, P. (1971). 'Electronic aids to night vision.' *Phil. Trans. R. Soc.* (A), **269**, 233–263
13 BERSON, E.L., MAHAFFLEY, L. and RABIN, A.R. (1974). 'A night vision pocketscope for patients with retinitis pigmentosa.' *Archs Ophthal.,* **91**, 6, 495
14 DUKE-ELDER, W.S. (1964). *System of Ophthalmology,* III, 2, 'Congenital Deformities.' p. 659. London: Kimpton
15 CARR, R.E., RIPPS, H., SIEGEL, I.M. and WEALE, R.A. (1966). 'Rhodopsin and the electrical activity of the retina in congenital night blindness.' *Investig. Ophthal.,* **5**, 497–507

Further reading

JAYLE, G.E., OURGAUT, A.G., BAISINGER, L.F. and HOLMES, W.J. (1959). *Night Vision.* Springfield, Illinois: Thomas

Chapter 10

Visual phenomena in the absence of correlating external stimuli

'. . . like a lot of flickering lights out of the corner of my eye.'

Visual sensations or perceptions occurring without a correlating external visual stimulus are termed hallucinations. They must be distinguished from visual illusions (*see* page 106). Visual hallucinations may be unformed (simple, primitive, elementary) or formed (complex).

Patients report many forms of visual experience independent of real visual stimuli in the environment. These vary from simple sensations of light and muscae to complex and sometimes grotesque hallucinations. The former may be of no consequence apart from annoyance to the individual or they can be the forerunner of disease. When the complexity of the eye's optical system, the intricacies of the retina and visual pathways and the ramifications within the brain resulting in perception are considered, it is little wonder that stimuli arising in the individual sometimes project themselves into consciousness, signalling, in some cases, an abnormal activity or unhealthy state. The related phenomena of chromatopsia, metamorphopsia and acquired dyschromatopsias are considered elsewhere in this work.

Formed hallucinations

Formed hallucinations consist of shapes, forms, patterns, people, animals or, in gross cases, crowds, armies and swarms of animals, sometimes advancing, sometimes receding, sometimes diminishing to minute size, but always giving a visual field full of activity. These bizarre experiences may be accepted calmly, they may equally cause great alarm. Few of the grosser cases of formed hallucinatory experience trouble the ophthalmic practitioner in the first instance for they arise in conditions where the patient will have sought or have been taken for investigation and treatment. They occur in some forms of blindness if the patient has previously been a seeing individual and may be very disturbing. They are also found in delirium, epilepsy, temporal lobe lesions, drug intoxication, gross mental disorders and in other neurological conditions.

Formed hallucinations of a non-alarming form can be precipitated in normal individuals after carrying out some exacting visual function for long periods. An example occurs in a visual task such as searching for, and picking, small fruit, such as blackberries. After several hours of this activity, most people experience a variety of distinctly formed hallucinations projected on to ordinary objects and scenes, particularly where the scene is reasonably flat and devoid of detail, such as a plain ceiling or wall. They are more vividly 'seen' when the eyes are closed. The impressions vary constantly; berries, leaves, buds and flowers in a never-ending display.

The ophthalmic practitioner might rarely have this type of experience reported during a history/symptom interview. Provided there are no significant symptoms or signs of neurological concern, and the history confirms the preceding visual task, then the patient can be reassured.

Unformed hallucinations

Unformed hallucinations are described in very many ways including flashes of light, rays of light, spots, sparks, zig-zags, scintillations, lightning flashes, coloured lights, balls of fire, coloured balloons, and white streaks. The most common causes include irritation of the retina in some form and irritation or stimulation of the occipital cortex as, for example, in migraine. Some of these will now be discussed.

Photopsia *(Table 10.1)*

The patient whose main symptom is that of flashes of light or sparks appearing in their visual field presents a problem, as with many similar symptoms, to which the answer may be exceedingly simple and of no significance clinically, or it may be an indicator of some serious eye condition.

TABLE 10.1. Causes of the Presenting Symptoms of Photopsia

Entoptic effects (for example, phosphenes, gravitational or 'blow' phenomenon)
Migraine
Adverse effects of drugs[10]
Retinal, choroidal and optic nerve conditions
Occipital cranial lesions, other than migraine
Epilepsy

Flashes of light may be complained of as a gravitational phenomenon or as a shock effect. Many will have experienced the white specks moving along circuitous paths which appear in the central field after bending down then straightening up rapidly. This kind of experience also happens frequently in some sporting occurrence, such as after the shock effect of topping a golf ball. Transient anaemia of the mascular vessels in which single corpuscles in the minute arterioles give rise to a visual stimulus is the usual explanation. The 'blow on the eye' phenomenon is well known for its sparks and light flashes and for its subsequent traction phosphenes, these also resulting from the mechanical effect on the retina.

Vascular spasm, arteriosclerosis and other vascular conditions in older patients are other causes of photopsia.

Photopsia of impending retinal detachment (separation)

The presenting symptom of light flashes is so emphasized in its relationship to predetachment that it is worth emphasizing that flashing lights or sparks, as described by the patient, are not pathognomonic of predetachment of the retina, although any such symptom must alert the examiner to that possibility. If the main symptom is one of photopsia, never having occurred before, with no subsequent headache, even if there is no description of other visual effect, then the probability of some irritative retino-choroidal lesion must be considered[1].

Photopsia, in the case of retinal detachment, are usually described in terms of arcs or flashes of white or coloured light, most noticeable on moving the eyes, transient at first, then becoming more persistent. They may be projected into a particular spatial direction and, if the upper retina detaches, appear in the lower part of the field. The moment of separation may be described by the patient as a 'cloud' or 'shower' of sparks or floaters. Visual loss is gradual and the patient often uses the description of a 'veil' or 'cloud' floating across the field of vision, usually from below.

Optometrists, rightly, become concerned about the patient who complains of photopsia, especially if this is the main symptom, and refer the patient even if there are no other suspicious signs at that stage. A history of trauma, which may be quite minor and a myopic refraction are additional indicators, but it must be remembered that isolated lighting flashes occur in myopia[3a] and in other patients without detachment of the retina[2,3a] and may be associated with vitreous separation. If the detached area approaches the macular area then central or paracentral metamorphopsia may be an additional symptom.

The detection of retinal detachment at as early a stage as possible is of very great concern to optometrists[3b] because it is a condition which demands urgent treatment, yet its incidence in general practice is not high. An extremely valuable method which is also rapid and simple is a nine-point observation technique of the retinal reflex from a distance of 40–60 cm[4]. This method is briefly described below in view of retinal detachment being one of the conditions in which the earlier its detection and treatment the more likely is the patient to retain useful vision.

Nine-point observation of the fundus reflex at 40–60 cm

In this method[4] the ophthalmoscopic reflex is examined in the nine principal directions of gaze at a distance of around 50 cm or further (*Figure 10.1*). The patient may be asked to move his eyes in the required directions, or greater control can be obtained if the patient fixes straight ahead and the examiner moves. The upper lids may have to be raised by hand in the latter case. Some ophthalmoscopes have a circular patch large enough to cover both pupils and a simultaneous comparison may be made of the twin reflexes. If this is done it must be remembered that pigmentation may differ in the quadrants, which will be nasal in one eye and temporal in the other. Most retinoscopic beams can be similarly used. Where the retina proper has lost, or begun to lose, its intimate adhesion to the pigment epithelium, a 'greying out' of the normal red reflex occurs, and this is very evident even at a very early stage of disturbance.

This change in quality of the reflex is much more difficult to observe with an ophthalmoscope used at the customary few centimetres for direct ophthalmoscopy. In this case the intensity of light escaping from the pupil and entering the sighthole overwhelms the subtle change in reflex, whereas at the larger distance minor changes in that reflected light are readily observed with the smaller angular subtense of the ophthalmoscopic sighthole.

Methods of detection for early retinal detachment

The following indicators assist in the investigation of possible early retinal detachment.

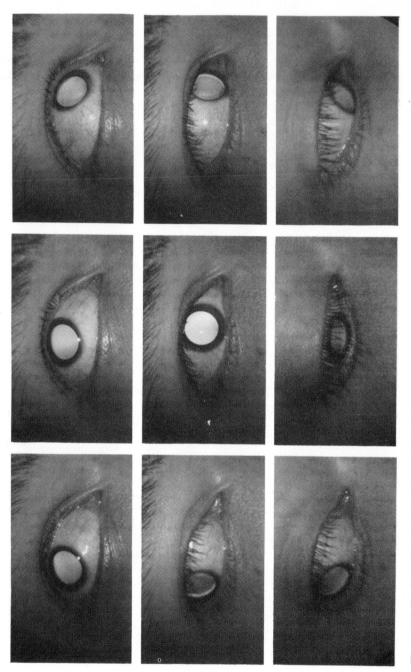

Figure 10.1. Fundus reflex in the nine diagnostic directions of gaze used for observation of changes in the quality of reflected light

History and symptoms History of trauma, myopia, aphakia; photopsia, floaters, central or paracentral metamorphopsia, unsteadiness of objects in space.

Ophthalmoscopic examination Nine-point observation of fundus reflex at 40–60 cm. Greying out of reflex in some direction of observation. Loss of retinal vascular reflexes, darkening of retinal vessels, retinal oedema, blurring of choroidal vessels. Greater positive power needed for clear ophthalmoscopic view. The later, very obvious, fundus changes are not dealt with here.

Photopsia in migraine

About 30–40 per cent of individuals suffering from migraine experience visual hallucinatory symptoms (visual aura) as an early indicator of an impending attack. In describing their visual experience patients use phrases such as: '. . . flickering lights out of the corner of my eye . . . like zig-zag or lightning flashes . . . dancing lights . . . shimmering . . .'

The initial visual symptom is commonly a very small flickering disturbance adjacent and to one side of the fixation point. This has been described by one of the author's patients as being 'like a tiny squirming transparent insect wriggling about just to the side of where I am looking.'

The flickering area expands slowly and colours appear within the flicker when it has developed to 15–25 degrees from the point of fixation. After 20 minutes or so the flickering area reaches the edge of the visual field and the form is lost in a vague assortment of greying flashes which then escape from the field altogether. The zig-zag pattern forms have been given the technical description of 'teichopsia' and 'fortification spectrum'.

To the central side of the flickering edge a hemianopic loss occurs and this lost area varies considerably with the individual and in individual attacks. Sometimes it merely shades away from the angular flashing pattern within a few degrees leaving the rest of the field quite normal. At other times the lost area recedes much less slowly than the expanding flashes so that a substantial hemianopic scotoma can be plotted. The subsequent headache also shows considerable variation both in intensity and location, although it is nearly always frontal and often contralateral to the temporary field defect.

Entoptic phenomena

Entoptic phenomena derive from the eye structures which have perceptive correlates projected into the visual field. Entoptic phenomena are not strictly hallucinations insomuch as a pre-receptor stimulus exists but it is present within the eye or on the corneal surface. Patients sometimes become alarmed when a simple entoptic observation is brought to their attention by some freak of viewing conditions. Examples occur in sunbathing when looking at a bright sky, or in semi-darkness, lying in bed gazing at a dimly illuminated ceiling. In the first case conditions are right for viewing muscae, in the second for becoming aware of the foveal scotoma of dim illumination (*Figures 10.2–10.5*). Entoptic effects have been thought to explain some reports of unidentified flying objects and it is true that entoptic observations, to the uninitiated, could wrongly be attributed to phenomena in the real world.

Discussion of entoptic effects is restricted to those most likely to be reported by patients during eye examination.

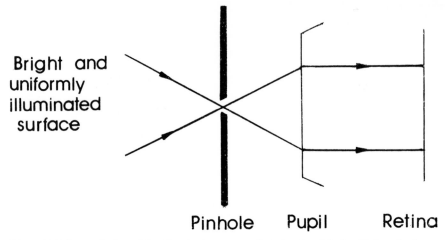

Figure 10.2. One optical condition for viewing muscae. Rotating the pinhole will show the fovea and foveal vessels (*see* also *Figure 10.5*)

'Floaters' and related observations

'. . . like little strings of beads floating in front of my vision'

The term floaters is usually interpreted as indicating opacities in the vitreous humour. This is often true but sometimes they merely delineate regions of different refractive index, as in muscae, rather than being true opacification. Because the patient describes them as floating need not locate them with certainty in the vitreous humour. Some patients use the word 'float' in the sense that the image moves as they move their eyes and a positive scotoma, although stationary in relation to the fixation point, moves around with the point of gaze.

Areas of greater or lesser refractive index most frequently result from remnants of the fetal hyaloid system and those which are seen and described clearly by the patient under normal viewing conditions lie close to the retina. They are best observed at high and under uniform levels of retinal illumination such as occur when gazing at a bright sky, a light wall or when using optical instruments like microscopes or telescopes (*Figure 10.3*).

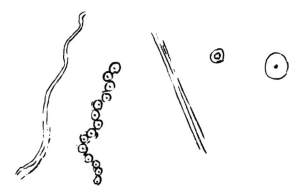

Figure 10.3. Types of muscae

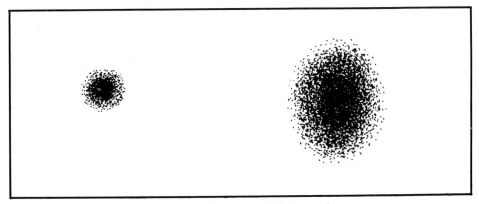

Figure 10.4. Vague and ghostly projections of macula and blind spot when viewing a uniformly grey surface on waking, under mesopic conditions. F = foveal-macular region. BS = blind spot

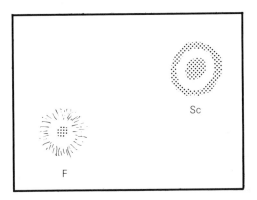

Figure 10.5. Retinal depigmented area observed entoptically through a rotating pinhole (*see also Figure 12.1* on page 121). F = fovea. Sc = scotoma

Opacities situated in the anterior vitreous humour reduce retinal illumination and may give spurious image formation in normal vision. Any visual effect is more noticeable when they lie near to the visual axis. They can be viewed by the patient under conditions suitable for entoptic observation (*Figure 10.2*). True floaters, rather than muscae are usually inflammatory, traumatic or degenerative in origin. Patients have many ways of describing muscae, amongst the most common being: strings of beads, threads, bubbles or globules, whisps of cotton, moving strands, spots, and all float downwards and the patient 'can't catch up with them'. Neurotic and hypersensitive patients complain most frequently, so do myopes and patients who are under some form of stress or fatigue. Practitioners should never bring these normal muscae to the attention of any patient who has not already reported them. Muscae are often mistaken for dust particles on the optical components of binoculars microscopes or telescopes. Dust on instrument lenses or prisms can, of course, be distinguished by remaining stationary but rotating with deliberate rotations of the various optical components.

The conventional wisdom in the case of muscae advises — if the patient can see them and the examiner cannot (by objective observation) then they are of no clinical significance. Although these assertions often accord with good practice there can

TABLE 10.2. Causes of Floaters

Non-pathological embryonic remnants
Myopia
Separation or adhesion of vitreous humour (shrinkage retraction)
Fluidity of vitreous humour
Vitreous haemorrhage
Retinal detachment
Uveitis
Foreign bodies (mostly in posterior vitreous humour except under special viewing conditions)

Note: Asteroid bodies (asteroid hyalitis) and synchisis scintillans rarely give rise to the symptom of floaters. Where the complaint of floaters appears to indicate a sudden origin or sudden rapid increase then some condition such as retinal separation must be suspected.

always be exceptions and the examiner should beware of adopting this rule as a *modus vivendi* in all cases. For example, as has been noted earlier, it very much depends on what the patient means by descriptions such as 'floating spots' and this must always be investigated. For a list of causes of floaters *see Table 10.2.*

Coloured halos around lights

Normal causes

Environmental   White lights seen through steamy windows at night appear to be surrounded by coloured rings. These rings may also be observed when looking at street lights through misted or frosted windscreens (windshields) of cars. This diffraction phenomenon is akin to the glaucomatous halo which is being 'seen' through an oedematous cornea.

Physiological[5]   The radial nature of the crystalline lens fibres causes a diffraction halo to be seen occasionally by the normal individual. The outer, red part of this normal halo subtends about 7–8 degrees.

Features distinguishing the various forms of halo

It is possible to distinguish between physiological-type and glaucomatous-type halos by their optical characteristics[6]. The observations needed are difficult enough for the experienced observer and results for untrained patients may therefore be inconclusive. The differentiation is based on the angular size of the halo and the effect of passing a narrow slit aperture across the pupil (*Table 10.3*).

TABLE 10.3. Distinguishing Features of Two Types of Subjective Halo[6]

	Angular size	Effect of narrow slit
Pathological (resulting from subacute angle closure glaucoma) (*Figure 10.6*)	Subtends more than 8 degrees	Halo remains intact but diminishes in intensity as slit passes over pupil
Normal (physiological)	Subtends less than 8 degrees	Halo disappears in part as slit passes over pupil

Pathological causes

The importance of avoiding suggestion in the questioning of susceptible patients has been noted earlier but it is worth re-emphasizing.

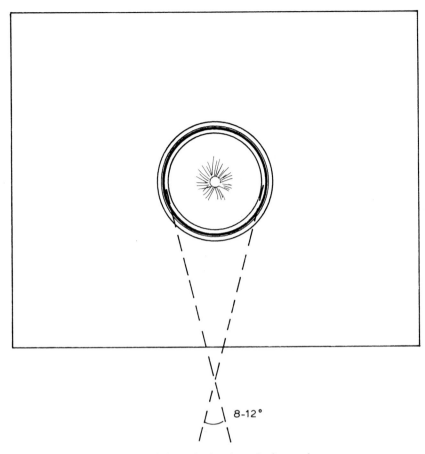

Figure 10.6. Glaucomatous-type halo as in chronic angle closure glaucoma

Sometimes a direct question on halos has to be asked if the information can neither be obtained spontaneously nor by indirect probing, but such a question as: 'Do you see coloured halos around white lights at night?' has to be used with care lest the neurotic patient or the patient wishing to please, readily agree and thereby despatch the examiner on roads of investigation all of which prove negative. The response to indirect questioning should be explored first by asking, for example, whether anything unusual has been noticed about white lights seen at night.

Coloured halos are complained of mostly in the subacute angle closure form of glaucoma and in framing the questions for the defined data of the history and symptom interview the prevalence of this kind of condition must be taken into account*.

Estimates of the incidence of subacute angle closure glaucoma vary between approximately 0.2 and 0.4 per cent. Chronic simple, or open angle glaucoma has a

---

*Two types of halo are described in glaucoma — an objective one and a subjective one. The subjective halo is described here. The objective halo is seen around the optic disc in the later stages of primary glaucoma.

much higher incidence of around 2–4 per cent of individuals over the age of 40–50 years[7,8,9].

Consider the case of a practitioner in general ophthalmic practice who sees 2,500 patients each year who might be at risk from such conditions. The numbers of patients who are likely to have one of the two forms of glaucoma is shown in *Table 10.4*.

TABLE 10.4. Probable Numbers of Patients Seen Each Year who have One of the Two Forms of Glaucoma Shown, From a Risk Population of 2500

Open angle glaucoma		Subacute angle closure glaucoma	
Approximate incidence		Approximate incidence	
2%	4%	0.2%	0.4%
50	100	5	10

If every patient is presented with a question about coloured halos in the history and symptom interview, then because the appearance is restricted almost entirely to the chronic angle closure variety, 2500 questions will be asked of the risk population with an expected negative response to at least 2490 of those questions. The examiner must consider such probabilities in the apportioning of skilled time. It is better for clinical experience to dictate and precipitate that kind of question based on an assessment of the individual patient's responses and on the ongoing data accruing in the subsequent examination. Alternatively, a questionnaire-type data-gathering process can be used by less skilled personnel, although this is not attractive to many patients who prefer the more personal approach of communication direct with the practitioner.

The glaucomatous halo should become apparent to the patient when the cornea is oedematous; indeed, any other condition causing corneal oedema is likely to precipitate a complaint of coloured halos. A complaint of coloured halos around lights at night, must not, therefore, be considered pathognomonic of some form of glaucoma. It could be a normal appearance (*see* above), but this symptom presented spontaneously by a patient must be treated with suspicion and investigated promptly. Problem-specific questions must be directed to determining the conditions under which halos are noticed — their frequency, whether transient, and whether other symptoms of subacute angle closure glaucoma occur such as transient blurring of vision (*q.v.*), headache (*q.v.*), ocular discomfort or pain (*q.v.*), and the time of day at which symptoms occur.

Chronic (simple) open angle glaucoma is not frequently associated with the halo symptom, nor with major symptoms at all, hence its insidious progress, quite unknown to the patient until a fairly late stage. For that condition there is a very special responsibility on the examiner, particularly in view of the higher incidence. The usual methods, including tonometry, visual field screening and ophthalmoscopic examination must be applied.

Phosphenes

In a somewhat darkened room, viewing conditions are right for the observation of phosphenes and sensitive patients may report these normal phenomena to the examiner. A quick eye movement produces traction on the optic nerve head and on the insertions of the extraocular muscles. The mechanical effect manifests itself as flashes of light projected into the respective parts of the visual field, often as a bright halo in

TABLE 10.5. Types of Entoptic Phenomena

Phosphenes
Lightning flashes
Muscae
Halos
Effects of the eye's aberrations
Retinal effects, for example, Haidinger's brushes, blue arcs, observation of retinal vessels, blind spot,
    fovea

the blind spot area. The colours experienced are usually yellow, violet and blue. After a blow on the eye a patient may report the continuous observation of traction phosphenes in a darkened room resulting from the disturbance to the muscle attachments and around the optic nerve head. These must be distinguished from the light flashes of impending retinal detachment. Only very careful questioning of the patient and objective examination will allow this distinction to be made (*Table 10.5*).

Pressure phosphenes are less likely to be presented as a problem by patients.

Aberrations

Spherical aberration

The most common observation connected with spherical aberration, and known to all those involved in visual science, is that distant objects appear to move 'with' the movements of the hand when looking through a very narrow gap (1–2 mm) between two of the fingers, demonstrating the usual positive spherical aberration at that fixation distance. Near objects tend to move against the movement of the gap, showing a change to negative spherical aberration. It is interesting to try to find the distance at which the point of reversal, or no movement, takes place.

Chromatic difference of magnification

This well-known phenomenon results in the apparent displacement forwards of red objects and is particularly obvious when looking at colour transparencies with the aid of a small viewer. Patients sometimes notice and comment on this appearance when viewing bichromatic (red-green) charts which have black characters seen on the coloured backgrounds. The effect depends on binocular viewing and it is useful and amusing to have a slide viewer in the consulting room office and to point out to patients how the red objects sink back into the flat landscape when one eye is closed. Colour slides when projected using a reasonable 'throw' to the screen, lose any false stereopsis due to chromatic difference of magnification.

Subjective effects connected with the pupil

The reduction in pupil diameter with age causes difficulty for older people in attempting to read in lighting conditions which in youth would be quite satisfactory. Miosis following the use of drugs gives the same effect. Higher illumination, together with the usual presbyopic addition, if needed, reduces the problem. In younger people the reduction in retinal illumination occurring during excessive accommodation and resulting from synergic pupil contractions is noticeable in dim illumination. Sometimes this is the only explanation to be offered for a patient's complaint that objects occasionally become dim as a transient phenomenon and then, only following very many and time-consuming investigations, all yielding normal results.

One effect of a large pupil is that a narrow gap between the fingers, held close to the eye, appears to coalesce as the fingers are brought even closer together, and shows typical changes as the gap is moved over the pupil, due to the grossly de-focused nature of the retinal image (*Figure 10.7*). These kinds of quite normal appearance may come to the attention of patients who work with optical devices involving small apertures.

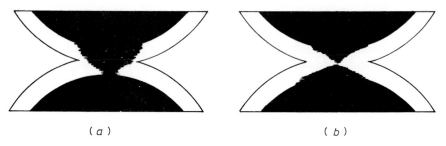

(*a*)   (*b*)

Figure 10.7. Apparent coalescing of fingertips as the slit aperture between them is further narrowed. (*a*) Aperture towards top of pupil. (*b*) Aperture centrally placed

Visual illusions

Although visual illusions occur in the presence of a stimulus in the environment, they are conveniently dealt with here.

A visual illusion occurs when the physical characteristics of an external stimulus are not reflected in the visual perception. The lay term for these effects is usually 'optical' illusion, but that description should be retained for illusions which are brought about by optical conditions such as mirages or where the effect is produced by optical devices.

Few of the common visual illusions are reported spontaneously by patients although they will sometimes mention optical illusions such as occur in heat haze (shimmering ground) or in driving (mirage effect of water on the road). Of the multitude of visual illusions and other related phenomena illustrated in works on psychology and visual science, those which rarely might be mentioned by patients are as follows.

Moon illusion. Apparent enlargement of the moon when near to the horizon.

Railroad illusion. The apparent motion of one's own stationary train as that on the adjacent platform moves out of the station.

Stroboscopic effect. The apparent slowing down or reversal of rotating objects seen on the cinema screen, especially the wheels of wagons in Western movies.

Illusion of motion after viewing motion. After looking at moving objects for a time, stationary objects then appear to creep slowly in a direction opposite to the previously observed movement.

Shadow illusion. Moon craters in photographs or similar objects appear as 'humps' rather than as depressions if the direction of illumination is misjudged.

All are normal effects and the patient can be reassured.

References

1 MORSE, P.H., SCHEIE, H.G. and AMINLARI, A. (1974). 'Light flashes as a clue to retinal disease.' *Archs Ophthal.*, **91**, 179–180
2 MOORE, R.F. (1935). 'Subjective lightning streaks.' *Br. J. Ophthal.*, **19**, 545–547
3a DUKE-ELDER, W.S. (1949). *Textbook of Ophthalmology*, Vol. IV, p. 3696. London: Kimpton
3b NATHAN, J. (1980). 'Referral criteria for pre-detachment disease.' *Aust. J. Optom.*, **63**, 19, 23
4 AMSLER, M. (1949). 'Detachment of the retina.' In *Diseases of the Eye*, p. 627, Ed. by BERENS, C. Philadelphia: Saunders
5 MELLERIO, J. and PALMER, D.A. (1970). 'Entoptic halos.' *Vis. Res.*, **10**, 7, 595–599
6 EMSLEY, H.H. (1952). *Visual Optics*, Vol. 1, p. 421. London: Butterworth
7 TREVOR-ROPER, P.D. (1974). *The Eye and its Disorders*, p. 530. Oxford: Blackwell
8 GRADLE, H.S. (revised by DUKE-ELDER, W.S.) (1949). 'Glaucoma.' In *Diseases of the Eye*, p. 579, Ed. by BERENS, C. Philadelphia: Saunders
9 COCKBURN, D.M. and GUTTERIDGE, I.F. (1980). 'Reasons for referral by optometrists to ophthalmologists: an audit of ocular disease detection.' *Aust. J. Optom.*, **63**, 13–18
10 ROY, F.H. (1975). *Ocular Differential Diagnosis*, p. 536. Philadelphia: Lea and Febiger

Further reading

CHANDLER, P.A. and GRANT, W.M. (1979). *Glaucoma*, 2nd ed. Philadelphia: Lea and Febiger
HEILMAN, K. and RICHARDSON, K.T. (Eds) (1978). *Glaucoma: Conceptions of a Disease.* Philadelphia: Saunders

Chapter 11

Discomfort in or around the eyes

'. . . I get a sharp pain behind my eyes.'

Sometimes referred to as *ocular* symptoms, discomfort in or around the eyes can have a very wide variety of causes, many of which are inconsequential but some of which are serious. In the absence of obvious signs, such as marked inflammation, it gives the greatest satisfaction to the practitioner when the cause can be identified. At the one extreme, discomfort arises from minor stress responses to life situations, and at the other by conditions such as early angle closure glaucoma. With many possible causes, including ametropia and binocular vision anomalies, how is the conscientious practitioner to proceed without becoming either confused or hypercautious to the extent of despatching each patient presenting this symptom for further investigations through specialist services? It would be simple to do so, at the expense of a catastrophic demand on those services, to the detriment of the majority of such patients in whom there can be no reasonable suspicion of eye, or eye manifestations of, general disease and to the detriment of the practitioner as a clinician.

Herein lies the essence of clinical decision making.

Where the aetiology is obscure, the responsibility is to form an opinion on the basis of the data collected during the history and symptom interview and in the following eye examination as to whether the discomfort is most likely to be arising from refractive, binocular vision or related anomalies or from other causes. These other causes will often be conditions with which the practitioner is conversant and experienced — high incidence anomalies or conditions on which emphasis has been placed by the health care concerns of the time. In other cases, usually the lower incidence conditions, an opinion can be formed only that there is a need for more highly specialized investigations.

The following guidelines do not set out to mimic standard texts in ophthalmology or general medicine. A full account of many of the conditions referred to in *Table 11.1* will be found in those works together with the diagnostic indicators. This applies also, with force, to the differentiation of superficial from deep injection of the conjunctival vessels.

Nevertheless, to avoid the reader being ensnared in a surfeit of named conditions, some indicators will be provided for clinical decision making in such patients.

Patients' descriptions of their discomfort

Patients whose eyes feel uncomfortable and who may or may not show conjunctival hyperaemia, voice their complaints in many different ways. Rarely do they say simply:

TABLE 11.1. Some Possible Causes of the Main Symptom of Discomfort In or Around the Eyes

WHITE EYE(S)		RED EYE(S)
With no significant hyperaemia in uncomplicated cases	*With superficial hyperaemia in uncomplicated cases*	*With marked hyperaemia superficial and/or deep*
Minor psychological stresses	Irritants	Loose or embedded foreign body
Use of eyes in prolonged exacting visual tasks	Lack of sleep	Corneal abrasions
Ametropia, presbyopia	Climate: cold, wind, sun	Conjunctivitis: chronic/acute in its many forms
Binocular vision anomalies	Contact lenses	Allergies
Sinus/nasal problems	Ametropia, presbyopia	Excess exposure to ultraviolet radiation
Contact lenses	Binocular vision anomalies	Sinus/nasal infections
Glaucoma — open angle (often symptomless)	Eyelash in punctum or in conjunctival sac	Other corneal afflictions: ulceration, keratitis
Early retrobulbar neuritis	Other minor foreign bodies	Trauma
Glaucoma — chronic angle closure	Allergies including conjunctival mucus (as in hay fever)	Blepharitis: chronic/acute in its many forms
Hysteria	Pinguecula	Acute iridocyclitis
Malingering	Styes	Infections of lacrimal apparatus
	Reduction in tear flow or lack of fluid reaching conjunctival sac	Acute glaucoma
	Minor trauma	Scleritis and episcleritis
	Sinus/nasal infections	Tumours
	Concretions	Malingering
	Trichiasis	
	Glaucoma — chronic angle closure	
	Nutritional deficiencies	
	Malingering (self-administered drugs/chemicals)	

Subconjunctival haemorrhage (commonly without discomfort)

'Dry' eye(s)
{
Age changes
Allergies
Toxins, drugs
Anomalies of lacrimal/conjunctival glands
Some forms of conjunctivitis
Nutritional deficiencies
Infrequent blinking
Some systemic diseases[9]
Rare syndromes[7]
}

Note: Discomfort may, or may not, be described in terms of 'pain' (*see* page 110).

'My eyes feel uncomfortable,' but add some word or words which seem most descriptive of their experience.

'My eyes feel . . . strained, heavy, tired, tight, stiff, hot, cold, itchy, dry, sandy, gritty, sticky, tacky, tender, delicate.'

Or: 'My eyes are . . . drawing, pulling, twitching, bloodshot, red, watery.'

None of these descriptions suggests real pain; the impression is one of more, or less, discomfort. Patients complain of having to shut or rub their eyes to gain temporary relief. Sometimes the description indicates a more painful sensation as in: 'My eyes are . . . sore, aching, smarting, burning, stinging.' Often the word 'pain' itself is used as in: 'I get a pain behind my eyes after I have been reading for some time.' And adjectives are added such as: 'gnawing pain, sharp pain, dull pain,' and so on.

These descriptions are more personality dependent than diagnostically significant but it is useful to record the words used by the patient as an indicator to psychological make-up and for possible use in any subsequent report. The degree of superficial conjunctival hyperaemia is an unreliable guide to the magnitude of the symptoms. This patient will live contentedly with minor injection, whilst another will stress the profound discomfort from a similar degree of injection. It can puzzle the student commencing clinical studies how it is that patients with marked chronic superficial conjunctival hyperaemia do not complain. Certainly, in some patients, increased secretion from the lacrimal or conjunctival glands may account for lack of symptoms but personality and adaptation to the chronic condition also play a role.

Neurotic and flamboyant subjects are prone to use extravagant expressions in describing their life experiences, just as much in the consulting room office as in their other human contacts. Where a patient uses extreme analogies in presenting symptoms one must suspect a neurotic temperament. Often these take the form of something rather horrible being done to their eyes or to their head: '. . . a sickening, boring pain right through my eyes from back to front as though a sharp knife were being pushed in deeper and deeper and twisted around.' The pain seems violent, akin to a clinical emergency such as acute glaucoma, but a single glance as the patient arrives through the consulting room office door is sufficient to discount that or similar conditions.

Patients should therefore be observed very closely for attitude and bearing as they answer questions as some indicator to the degree of discomfort from which *the practitioner* assesses them to be suffering — this to rank alongside the patient's own account.

Questioning the patient

Simple, problem-oriented questions are presented to probe the complaint of discomfort, as follows.

Type	'Can you describe exactly how your eyes feel?'
Onset, course	'When did you first notice the problem?'
and	'Has it remained the same or varied?'
Relationships	'Is it worse at any time of day?' 'Does the discomfort come on when you are involved in any particular job or activity?'

Unilateral—Bilateral	'Do both eyes seem to be affected?'
*Vision**	'What is your vision like out of doors and for reading?'
Presence of exudation	'Do you find that your eyelids stick together in the mornings?' 'Is there any discharge?'
Presence of photophobia	'Do bright lights or does daylight bother you?'
*Related symptoms**	'Have you noticed any other problems such as headache?'

Eye discomfort in small amounts of ametropia and minor binocular vision anomalies

Discomfort in and around the eyes (as distinguished from Visual Unease — *see* Chapter 6) is a very common experience in patients with small hypermetropic-type refractive errors, early presbyopia or low heterophoria, but it can also occur through stress or in other psychoneurotic states.

This kind of discomfort is sometimes described as 'eye strain' but the term is widely interpreted and loosely defined. It is a description rarely used by patients, but if so, the meaning attributed to it by the patient must be the subject of close questioning. It is considered by some[1] that eye pain, in the absence of inflammation, is very rarely attributable to any underlying disease.

Where only very small refractive and binocular vision errors are found, all other data are within normal expectations and mild eye discomfort is the sole presenting symptom, decision-making becomes much less certain. The history and symptom discussion then assumes greater significance. When the refractive and binocular vision findings have been determined, the symptoms must be reviewed by re-phrasing many of the earlier questions, preferably in indirect form, so that the patient neither appreciates the duplication nor is subject to undue suggestion. Check — re-check questioning often uncovers symptoms not previously remembered or reported — symptoms which can be crucial to the decision of whether or not to prescribe. The eye discomfort arising in small amounts of hypermetropia, hypermetropic astigmatism, early presbyopia or small degrees of heterophoria mirrors that in minor psychological stress and these conditions together account for the majority of patients voicing this complaint.

There is no formula yet devised which will advise the practitioner with certainty whether or not to prescribe in marginal cases of ametropia or heterophoria. In making these decisions much will depend on the problem-specific data for the individual patient rather than on the degree of ametropia or heterophoria. One practitioner will decide to prescribe for this patient, another will not, both acting genuinely and ethically according to their own tenets of good practice. The student of optometry will have conflicting advice in these marginal cases.

Nevertheless, if the examiner has a problem then so does the patient. In some patients with discomfort of obscure aetiology, the correction of apparently minor optical defects may be one step in the elimination of potential causes of that discomfort where previous measures have failed. If symptoms disappear, as they are likely to do for a time from the placebo effect, only their long-term absence will confirm the diagnosis. If symptoms recur in their original form then one must look elsewhere.

---

*Usually asked and answered earlier in the interview.

It would be valuable to have greater certainty in making borderline decisions and in the general decision-making process of prescribing optical corrections. There is a weight of experience to find its way into diagnostic data banks from which the probability of symptoms arising from defined patient data will be predictable. An assessment of probabilities is no substitute for decisions, but it will help the examiner, particularly if working single handed, to have the cumulative experience on hand for all types of prescribing situations.

Students and examinations

Students preparing for examinations show a marked increase in requests for eye examination[2]. Their complaints are mostly of eye discomfort with few visual symptoms. Eye examination, if carried out, reveals age-norm clinical emmetropia in most cases, with other functions within normal limits. Symptoms are as likely in the high flyer as in the potential failure.

Overwork, hurried meals and late nights head a long list of tension-producing life situations. Most of the complaints disappear soon after examinations are completed. Reassurance that there is no need for any optical correction, if that proves to be the case, gives some relief from the symptoms.

The possibility of anomalies of accommodation and convergence and the presence of oblique axis astigmatism related to the studies (*see* below) must be investigated but few prove to have such anomalies.

Low, positive-powered lenses, incorporating small base-in prisms, prescribed as a temporary measure for close work will probably be said by the patient to help, but it is likely that these act more as a gratefully accepted but clear placebo, rather than their optical properties having any significant effect in reducing symptoms. Where there are no indicators of abnormality it is far wiser to defer action until the stress of examinations has passed, and to avoid establishing cases of spectacle dependency.

Assessment

When assessing the probability of vague eye discomfort arising from low degrees of ametropia or heterophoria and therefore the necessity or otherwise for an optical prescription the following information must be taken into account.

(1) The apparent magnitude of the problem to the patient.

(2) Stress-producing life situations and general health judged from the history/symptom interview.

(3) The patient's age.

(4) The visual tasks being undertaken, critical detail, luminances, contrast, working conditions.

(5) Degree and type of ametropia or binocular vision anomaly and adaptation ability to that anomaly, especially to heterophoria.

(6) The effect of medication.

Special situations and task-related eye discomfort

(1) Low values of astigmatism which would not be expected to produce symptoms are annoying to a few hypersensitive patients whose work is visually exacting. Correction of such astigmatic errors relieves the discomfort but may introduce an element of distortion into the patient's visual environment for a time. This distortion is usually noticed and reported by that type of patient so that a mild warning of this possibility should be given at the initial examination. Small oblique-axis astigmatism is the usual offender.

(2) Workers using microscopes in their work often complain of discomfort and headaches and there are several possible causes. The discomfort may occur as a fatigue effect from continually closing one eye — usually the non-dominant one — in the use of monocular instruments. The patient should be encouraged to keep both eyes open and ignore the unwanted image. An incorrect focusing procedure also leads to problems where the work involves binocular microscopes or other binocular instruments. Excess accommodation is used or there is monocular blur and hence visual unease.

(3) Recent changes in the visual working environment trigger complaints of eye discomfort as during a change-over to fluorescent from other forms of lighting or in the use of visual display units. The problem is generally precipitated by operators who have manifest visual problems or by those showing stress in the new conditions, especially from the fear of so-called 'eye damage'. An hysterical-type group reaction can be generated amongst those working under the same conditions. The alleged guilty agency is revealed early in the history and symptom discussion; indeed, it is usually the first described and main symptom. Decisions on whether there is, or is not, a real visual working problem cannot be made in the isolation of the consulting room office and those decisions may involve the organizations responsible for the staff in the place of work. A study of the working environment and of the visual task together with personal discussions and examination of the operators is the only sure route to a long-term solution once such group problems have arisen.

All that can be done during normal eye examination is to correct significant optical or other errors based on good practice, taking into account the demands of the visual task as assessed from the patient's description and observations. Whether special prescriptions are desirable, whether changes in the working environment are needed, or whether general advice to the works management or staff ought to be given are matters which can be resolved only in liaison with those responsible for the place of work.

Visual tasks associated with this kind of response include many industrial devices, particularly visual display units[3,4], oscilloscopes, print magnifying devices, computer print-outs. Attention must be given to the positioning of the device, colour and contrast in the surroundings, ventilation, general luminance levels, acuity and vergence movements necessary for size and speed of presentation, age of the operator, operator's visual acuity, correction of ametropia, presbyopia, heterophoria.

(4) After prolonged driving, many complain of eyes feeling 'tight', 'taut' or 'stiff', together with a feeling of having to 'peer' or 'stare' to see properly. In the absence of significant refractive error or heterophoria the conditions of driving such as posture, rest periods, effective use of sun visors even in the absence of sun if the sky is bright, release of stress to external eye muscles by eye movements or rest (having regard to the safety of the vehicle), must be attended to.

These symptoms also arise in prolonged television viewing or in the cinema.

Attention must be given to the positioning of the television set preferably not above the horizontal, and to the reduction of screen contrast with that of the background.

Discomfort arising from a 'red' eye or eyes

The task of an optometrist or ophthalmic optician in general practice is simplified somewhat where discomfort is arising from an eye or eyes which are manifestly 'red'. The majority of patients who complain of gross eye irritation or pain and who have a red eye or eyes are unlikely to present themselves to such practitioners in the first instance unless there are special local or geographical situations. For patients who do happen to attend for examination in optometric practice, the immediate responsibility is to discuss the history, examine the patient and to form an opinion on the relative urgency with which the patient needs other than emergency attention. The normal procedure would then be to refer the patient for medical examination.

The red eye, as it is called (*see* below), has an array of causes and the practitioner cannot be aware of every rare syndrome which might be present. In general practice the most common cause of the red eye, usually with no discomfort, will be the result of subconjunctival haemorrhage; where there is discomfort, then foreign bodies in the conjunctival sac and minor corneal abrasions would rank high in probability, along with conditions such as some form of conjunctivitis or allergy. Unilateral subconjunctival haemorrhage presents a somewhat special problem in that — unless there is a history of trauma, or some other general or eye disease exists — it is usually of no significance[5].

It is common practice to write and talk about the red eye and its diagnostic significance and this simple description has been retained here, but with some reservation. There can be no doubting the redness in many acute states, but all variants may be encountered dependent on the condition and its progress, from minor discolorations to the fully blown redness of a recent and massive subconjunctival haemorrhage. Older texts described the violent redness of acute catarrhal conjunctivitis and then paradoxically referred to the condition as 'pink' eye, so, even in these serious deliberations, the practitioner may be excused a little artistic license.

'Dry' and 'watering' eyes

Because a patient's eye is clinically dry, in the objective sense, does not mean that the main symptom will be of a dry-feeling eye. More likely is itchiness or grittiness with some photophobia or any of the typical descriptions used by patients whose eyes are injected (*see* page 110). The symptom of tearing will be foremost in the history for patients with a watering eye and correlates with the objective appearance. Metamorphopsia (Chapter 12) and visual blur (Chapter 6) may be secondary symptoms.

A dry eye suffers from either diminished secretion of the conjunctival or lacrimal glands or, if secretion is normal, from lack of tear fluid reaching the conjunctival sac. A watering eye has either excessive tear production or proper drainage is being prevented.

Symptoms arising from dry or watering eyes are some of the most common in ophthalmic practice. The dry eye affects the patient primarily, but the watering eye provokes great distress both from the personal discomfort and embarrassment caused when in company with others.

The older patient is prone to both these conditions. Lacrimal secretion decreases as a normal ageing process[6] and discomfort occurs especially out of doors or in smokey atmospheres. Withdrawal of the punctum from close contact with the conjunctival sac prevents proper outflow of lacrimal fluid and hence epiphora. Normal individuals experience watering eyes in emotive situations and as an effect of wind, sun or cold; sometimes also from long exposure to sun and its attendant ultraviolet radiation, as in sunbathing (*Table 11.2*). The most frequent reason for a unilaterally watering (and red) eye is from a loose foreign body in the conjunctival sac but the practitioner must be alert to making assumptions solely because the patient reports something 'going into my eye'. There may well be a loose or embedded foreign body, but the discomfort is just as likely to arise from the resulting corneal abrasions long after the offending particle has been washed or rubbed out. Alternatively, the report of a foreign body may be mistaken or dissociated from the real condition causing the discomfort. The measures to be taken will depend on the rules or laws under which the optometrist practises.

TABLE 11.2. Causes of Watering Eyes

Cold, wind, sun (especially older patients)
Emotion, pain
Foreign body: loose, embedded
Corneal abrasion
Irritants (especially in industry) and allergies
Misplacement of punctum (especially older patients)
Ametropia, presbyopia, binocular vision anomalies
Conjunctivitis of some form
Other corneal afflictions, for example, ulceration
Lacrimal gland anomalies
Obstruction to tear drainage
Rare syndromes

Within these rules, the interests of the patient must be the first concern. The dry eye occurring in older patients from decreased lacrimal gland secretion is relieved somewhat by artificial tears, provided there are no other indicators to abnormal function. In these patients there should be close collaboration with the patient's general medical adviser. In suspected embedded foreign bodies, focal and fluorescein examination are pre-requisites to emergency action. Mild corneal anaesthesia may be necessary in marked blepharospasm if the cornea is to be examined and the upper lid everted.

Notes on special symptoms of discomfort

'Hot' and 'cold' eyes

The complaint of a hot or cold feeling in the eyes can arise in the same individual with the same condition but under different conditions. If the conjunctiva is injected, the eyes often feel hot when the lids are closed but cold when the lids are open. The coldness is more marked in the open air provided the air temperature is not too high.

These symptoms are most likely to occur in chronic conjunctival hyperaemia such as occurs in allergies, pingueculae and similar conditions including the effect of alcohol and insomnia.

Photophobia

The word photophobia indicates a fear of light, yet clinically it has become synonymous with discomfort and intolerance to light levels which would not normally be expected to provoke such a response. The word is often also confused with the less subjective condition of glare.

Obsessional photophobia of psychogenic origin in which a true fear of light exists is uncommon. The patient attempts to live in a world of semi-darkness or near darkness[1] and rarely will such a patient be seen in optometric practice. Nevertheless, mild, functional or psychic photophobia in which there appears to be patient discomfort to commonly encountered light levels, is a frequent symptom presented in the consulting room, and the guiding principle in the optometric management of photophobia must be to trace the cause and not to treat the symptom except as a temporary expedient to offer some relief to the patient.

The low level discomfort found in non-inflammatory conditions has to be differentiated from the gross discomfort, blepharospasm and marked intolerance to light where some inflammatory state exists. This latter, severe form of photophobia should not allow for misinterpretation, but the mild states have very diverse origins including functional causes as for the psychic photophobes mentioned above. *Table 11.3* suggests some of these causes. For example, those who have lived their lives in equatorial regions often show some mild discomfort in sunlight or to the natural sky light of higher latitudes, such as in Great Britian, yet not in their country of origin. This is strictly a glare problem which arises from the generally lower altitude of the sun through the day in higher latitudes. This gives greater values to the light and ultraviolet light directly incident and reflected from surfaces than the person has been accustomed to, particularly when involved in common activities such as driving.

TABLE 11.3. Some Causes of Photophobia

Generally mild	Hay fever
	Mydriasis from drugs and other causes
	Functional
	Corneal irritation (for example, foreign body in conjunctival sac)
	Contact lens wear
	Myopia
	Migraine
	Trigeminal irritability
	Post-operative aphakia
	Retrobulbar neuritis
	Anterior segment lesions (for example, keratoconjunctivitis, iridocyclitis, corneal ulceration, iritis)
	Toxins and adverse effects of drugs[8]
	Buphthalmos
Generally severe	Febrile conditions
	Partial or total aniridia
	Albinism
	Achromatopsia
	Obsessional psychogenic

References

1 DUKE-ELDER, W.S. (1949). *The Practice of Refraction,* 5th ed., p. 6. London: Churchill
2 BALL, G.V. and BOLTON, R.H. (1960–70). Unpublished data. Freshmen visual screening. University of Birmingham, England
3 HARLEN, F. (1978). 'Radiation: the non-hazard of V.D.U's.' In *Visual Aspects and Ergonomics of Visual Display Units,* Ed. by READING, V.M., pp. 101–107. London: Institute of Ophthalmology
4 MACKAY, C. (1980). 'Human factors aspects of visual display unit operation.' *H.S.E. Research paper* 10. London: H.M. Stationery Office
5 HAVENER, W.H. (1979). *Synopsis of Ophthalmology,* 5th ed., p. 268. St. Louis: Mosby
6 FURUKAWA, R.E. and POLSE, K.A. (1978). 'Changes in tear flow accompanying ageing.' *Am. J. Optom. physiol. Opt.,* **55,** 2, 69–74
7 NEMA, H.V. (1973). *Ophthalmic Syndromes,* pp. 240, 280. London: Butterworth
8 GREEN, H. and SPENCER, J. (1969). *Drugs with Possible Ocular Side-effects,* p. 187–192. New York: St. Martin's Press
9 THYGESON, P. (1951). 'Dermatoses with ocular manifestations.' In *Systemic Ophthalmology,* Ed. by SORSBY, A., pp. 586–587. London: Butterworth

Further reading

PAU, H. (Trans. CIBIS, G.) (1978). *Differential Diagnosis of Eye Disease.* Philadelphia: Saunders
ROY, F.H. (1975). *Ocular Differential Diagnosis.* Philadelphia: Lea and Febiger
TREVOR-ROPER, P.D. (1974). *The Eye and its Disorders.* London and Oxford: Blackwell

Chapter 12

Visual confusion and disturbances in space perception

'. . . and, suddenly everything seemed to go very small.'

Two general types of symptom are considered under the above heading: (1) metamorphopsia; and (2) faulty spatial localization.

Metamorphopsia*

Metamorphopsia — the various forms of which are listed in *Table 12.1* — describes the state of visual perception in which space or objects in space appear distorted. This distortion may be regular or irregular. Regular distortions include the following.

Micropsia (Lilliputian syndrome)   Objects appear abnormally small
Macropsia (megalopsia)   Objects appear abnormally large
Teleopsia   Objects appear abnormally far off
Pelopsia   Objects appear abnormally close
    The suffix 'varians' may be added to any of the above terms indicating that the effect varies during fixation, for example, micropsia varians.

Metamorphopsia occurring in normal individuals

Some forms of metamorphopsia are reported by normal patients.

Strong convergence/accommodation

If convergence and accommodation take place much in excess of that required for single clear vision of the object of regard then micropsia may be experienced. The convergence function may be the prime triggering mechanism for the apparent minification of objects, with accommodation playing a subsidiary role[1], but there is still some debate on the question. Changes in convergence may also change the receptive fields[2].

Teleopsia varians is a fairly common experience

In this condition objects retreat from the observer as though seen through a 'zoom' lens going from larger to smaller or vice versa, usually the former. It occurs when an individual becomes drowsy or following over-indulgence in alcohol or from the

---

*Some authorities[3] restrict the term metamorphopsia to visual distortion within the visual field. Here it is used in the more general sense of distortion within or of the whole visual field.

TABLE 12.1. Various Forms of Metamorphopsia

Metamorphopsia	Physiological, for example, strong accommodation/convergence Refractive Retinal Neurological Drugs, toxins [15]
Macropsia	Vision through hazy atmospheres Recently corrected presbyopia, hypermetropia Base-in prisms and other optical devices Spasm of accommodation
Micropsia	Vision in very clear atmospheres Base-out prisms and other optical devices Recently corrected myopia Neurosis, psychosis Intoxication Palsy of accommodation Occipital and parietal lobe lesions
Irregular metamorphopsia	Vision through prisms Media irregularities Central retinal oedema Macular degeneration Central lesions[16]
Teleopsia	Vision in hazy atmospheres In drowsiness (transient) Occipital and parietal lobe lesions Intoxication (varians) Neurosis, psychosis (usually transient)
Pelopsia	Recent optical corrections (for example, presbyopic additions) Vision in very clear atmospheres Neurosis, psychosis

misuse of drugs. In the latter cases the sensation of suddenly diminishing objects is accompanied by a nauseating sensation, relieved by closing the eyes. Sudden, uncontrolled convergence is the likely explanation.

Apparent movement of the visual world is another common experience

This occurs as an illusive effect from types of stimuli used in the vision science laboratory or after travelling for some time in one direction whilst observing the passing landscape, then stopping suddenly. Although this is an apparent movement of the environment rather than a direct enlargement or minification of objects, the slowly advancing or retreating landscape gives the sensation of increasing or decreasing size. The effect is best observed if the individual remains undisturbed and the visual field contains no moving objects.

Macropsia is a normal experience when looking through hazy atmospheres to those not used to such conditions

People and objects loom out of fog appearing larger than they should. A resident of Great Britain who has become accustomed to distant hills being seen through atmospheric haze, misjudges the distances and sizes of mountains at first when seen in very clear atmospheres, assessing them to be lower and nearer. Conversely, visitors to Great Britain from the clear air of mountainous regions often consider hills to be many thousands of metres higher and further away than they really are. In the clear air of mid-ocean, ships appear closer and smaller than around misty coasts, due to their sharper outlines[4].

A small degree of micropsia is evident to normal individuals when first looking through weak negative (concave) lenses

A large minification occurs when observing through the magnifying system of a reversed Galilean telescope. This is put to good use in peephole door devices or in field expanders for conditions such as the late stages of retinitis pigmentosa (*see* Chapter 9). The apparent paradox of a magnifying system which reduces the observed sizes of objects stems from the general definition of magnification as the ratio of image to object sizes. Apparent enlargement of objects both at distance and at near is produced by a multitude of simple and complicated optical devices varying from single convex lens hand magnifiers to the compound optical systems of microscopes and telescopes. Prismatic optical devices give a complex distortion of objects depending on the base position and direction of gaze through the prism.

Metamorphopsia in corrected ametropes who are otherwise normal

When ametropia is first corrected or following a change in prescription, spatial distortion is often complained of with the new lenses. Most patients adapt rapidly (Chapter 5).

The most frequent reason therefore for the presenting symptom of metamorphopsia, particularly for micropsia or macropsia, is the very optical prescription given to relieve some optical defect. The distorting effects of lenses arise from prismatic elements, differences in magnification between the two eyes, aberrations, and the impact on accommodation and convergence, as well as from any real change in retinal image size.

Newly corrected presbyopes notice apparent enlargement of reading matter although the actual enlargement of the retinal, compared to the normal, image is minimal if the lenses are fitting close to the eyes. Recently and fully corrected myopes complain of micropsia until adaptation takes place.

Newly corrected oblique astigmatism is well known to optometrists as a cause of temporary spatial distortion, and sometimes in a mistaken attempt to reduce possible distortion the cylinder axis is arbitrarily moved nearer to the horizontal or vertical, often with disastrous results from the resultant cylinder and residual axis meridian of the then obliquely crossed cylinders of eye and correcting lens.

These minor space distortions with optical corrections can often be demonstrated in the vision science laboratory by methods such as space eikonometry, but most never register in the patient's consciousness. If they do or in the more pronounced distortions then the patient may present tolerance problems which have to be handled carefully if the relationship between examiner and patient is to be preserved. These aspects are dealt with in Chapter 5.

Anomalies of accommodation and convergence

Metamorphopsia occurring in normal individuals as a result of changes in accommodation and convergence has already been mentioned and, likewise, abnormalities in the convergence/accommodation function can also give rise to regular metamorphopsia.

Palsy of accommodation/convergence gives micropsia; conversely, spasm results in macropsia. In the former case the patient has to make an abnormally strong effort in an attempt to obtain single and clear binocular vision. Because the visual angle of the object of attention remains constant, it is judged to be closer and therefore smaller.

Pathological metamorphopsia of peripheral origin

Retinal metamorphopsia attributable to retinal sensory element displacement

If, for some reason, the retinal sensory elements suffer distortion or displacement then the perceived image reflects that distortion or displacement most noticeably when the central region of the retina is affected at, or near to, the macula (*Figure 12.1*). Retinal distortion in the periphery usually passes unnoticed. Anything, therefore, which disturbs the positioning of the sensory endings may lead to the presenting symptom of metamorphopsia, most likely of the irregular form.

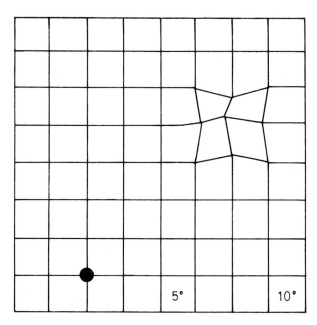

Figure 12.1 Irregular paracentral metamorphopsia. Grid distortion representing small retinal depigmented area following toxic disturbance. Fixation on spot (*see also Figure 10.5*)

Oedematous central retinal conditions: tumours, exudates, inflammations, cicatricial changes, macular degenerations, retinal detachment, all can prompt the symptom of metamorphopsia when affecting the central region of the retina as well as causing changes in visual acuity and other related symptoms and signs. If the abnormal retinal change causes the retinal cells to become crowded, then macropsia is to be expected: if they become greatly separated then micropsia is usual. Irregularity is common in the perceived image.

Notes on methods of examination

Because the complaint of metamorphopsia is most common when the central retinal region is affected, then line charts can be used to demonstrate the subjective appearance. The use of line charts in the investigation of metamorphopsia is ancient and referred to in several works in general ophthalmology[5]. Simple line charts can be constructed by the examiner to suit the individual mode of practice or the series of Amsler grid charts can be used[6]. It is, however, most unwise to stress these central visual distortions to patients by plotting and replotting their distribution or by using many different charts and methods of investigation. It is best if the patient learns to ignore the effects on vision[7] and is dissuaded from covering off one eye in order to judge regularly the extent of their defect. With minor disturbances the distortions are largely obscured in binocular viewing provided that the affected areas do not superimpose.

Pathological metamorphopsia of central origin

Hallucinogens such as cannabis indica or mescaline[8] produce marked visual effects including photopsia (Chapter 10): chromatopsia (Chapter 7) and sometimes metamorphopsia, usually of the microptic variety. Ethyl alcohol even in moderate quantities and in susceptible individuals, as has been mentioned earlier, can induce teleopsia and a feeling of dissociation from the real world. The visual world recedes suddenly, often accompanied by dizziness or true vertigo and a sensation of 'pulling' of the eyes — all probably arising from sudden, uncontrolled convergence movements. The grosser condition of toxic delirium is remarkable for its hallucinatory effects of coloured microptic animal and other forms, which with possible double vision are well-known symptoms even to the lay person. Intoxication from atropine and hyoscine has also been reported to lead to this kind of microptic hallucination[8].

Disturbances of the parietal and occipital lobes including tumours and trauma may precipitate micropsia and macropsia, usually the former. Micropsia is also experienced in migraine, epilepsy, neurosis and psychosis[8].

Irregular refractive metamorphopsia

Irregularities of the optical media, particularly of the anterior surface of the cornea, give rise to irregularities in the retinal image. Patients who are so affected may complain of metamorphopsia. Other symptoms may override this complaint, however, particularly that of reduced vision or monocular diplopia. Patients use many different ways of describing their visual irregularity: 'When I look at things they seem to be . . . shimmering . . . broken up . . . in fragments . . . bent . . . crooked.'

Corneal abnormalities which are most likely to cause metamorphopsia include pterygium and keratoconus. Senile-type cortical cataract, especially in its early stages is also a cause of possible irregularity in the perceived images. As for all types of metamorphopsia, the simple presenting symptom must be investigated by problem-oriented questions in the first place before proceeding to subjective and objective examination.

Faulty spatial localization

Although cerebral lesions are commonly associated with difficulties in spatial localization, a particular form occurs in paretic strabismus. In normal circumstances, the impulses to the extraocular muscles correspond to the angular rotations undertaken by those muscles. In pareses of an extraocular muscle the nervous impulse necessary for a certain action results in a lesser movement in the affected direction. In binocular conditions, diplopia would occur in the direction of action of the faulty muscle and this is the usual symptom in recent palsies. In time, a new head posture will be adopted to redistribute the remaining field of single binocular vision.

In monocular viewing by the affected eye, localization of objects in space will be faulty, demonstrated for example by past-pointing and other tests in the field of action of the muscle concerned. Rarely, a patient might notice problems when the other, unaffected eye is prevented, for some reason, from assuming its normal overriding function, for example, in accidental occlusion of the good eye, by some object in the environment. The usual complaint, however, will be of visual confusion due to diplopia and dizziness.

Visual confusion and vertigo

The term vertigo (*Table 12.2*) has two conventional interpretations: (1) A sense of continuing directional rotation of the body or of the environment (giddiness, severe or true vertigo); (2) A sensation resulting from loss of judgement of body position in space (dizziness — *Table 12.3,* mild vertigo).

Patients do not complain of vertigo unless they are well versed in medical matters. The usual description given by patients is that of feeling unsteady, dazed, a sense of spinning or whirling around, of staggering and being about to fall. If the body or surroundings appear to be rotating then the patient will be distressed, confused and probably complain also of nausea.

Dizziness, or vertigo defined as in (2) above, does not involve a sense of directional rotation and is experienced, for example, by many people when high up from the ground. Golfers playing from a high tee which shelves away steeply in front, experience a sense of weakness and dizziness, often described as vertigo, as though the body were about to be projected forward into space as the club is swung through the ball[9]. But this is not *true* vertigo. The term should be restricted to conditions where objects in space or the patient's body appear to be rotating in a particular direction — the form accompanied by jerky nystagmus, usually of vestibular or central origin. In

TABLE 12.2. True Vertigo (with Jerky Nystagmus and Subjective Directional Sense of Rotation)

Physiological, from artificial labyrinthine stimulation
Ménière's syndrome
Pathological nystagmus[17] of peripheral or central origin, for example:
    Acute labyrinthitis
    Lesions of vestibular pathways
    Raised intracranial pressure
    Multiple sclerosis
    Lesions of brain stem or cerebellum
    Vascular lesions
Adverse effect of drugs or toxins, for example, alcohol

TABLE 12.3. Dizziness (Mild Vertigo-type Sensations usually Without Nystagmus and With No Sense of Continuing Directional Rotation)

Effects of heights
Heterophoria and pareses of extraocular muscles
Recently corrected refractive errors causing spatial distortion
Some forms of bifocal and multifocal correction in susceptible patients
Circulatory problems as in fainting
Accommodation spasms
Metamorphopsia, refractive or retinal
Adverse effect of drugs[15]

objective vertigo the environment appears to be in a state of continual rotation. In *subjective* vertigo, the patient feels that the body is rotating.

True vertigo accompanied by the jerky form of nystagmus rarely arises from a primary ocular cause. Recently acquired jerky nystagmus produces gross confusion, incapacitation and nausea and it is most unlikely that such patients will present themselves for conventional eye examination with this as the main presenting symptom, although vertigo may be reported as part of the patient's history[10]. Vertigo-like complaints may be noted in the history/symptom interview and the exact nature of the complaint must be determined if this is possible at that stage. Usually these complaints prove to be a lesser or greater sense of dizziness with no directional rotation of either the body or the environment. One exception to this common experience is the report of vertigo from Ménière's syndrome[11]. Common in older males, medical attention has usually been received around the time of the attacks.

Pendular-type nystagmus is sometimes seen as a congenital condition or in cases where bilateral visual acuity is lowered at a very early age. Apparent movement of the environment and hence vertigo are not normally presenting symptoms in those conditions.

Vertigo occurring in normal individuals

Vertigo occurs normally with sudden changes in body position or rotation. The resulting nystagmus is best demonstrated when the rotation lies in the plane of one pair of semi-circular canals. It is common after some types of fairground ride. It is well known that dancers avoid vertigo and jerky nystagmus in pirouettes by retaining the head stationary for as long as possible, then rotating it rapidly back to the original position. When near to sleep, or in drowsiness, objects suddenly move jerkily downwards with increasing velocity and then are arrested as attention revives. This apparent vertical rotation of the environment, possibly associated with diplopia and blurring from relaxation of accommodation and convergence, is linked to Bell's phenomenon. Some normal people are able to induce voluntary nystagmus as a way of amusing friends[12].

It is a common experience that the jerky form of nystagmus occurs naturally if the environment itself is rotating or moving past the observer. The rotating drum stripes in nystagmography do not cause vertigo but lead to some discomfort for many patients although most can tolerate the experimental procedures without too much distress. Similarly, optokinetic, or railroad nystagmus induced by the moving scene seen from the railway carriage does not give rise to complaint unless the person has a type of heterophoria which becomes intermittently decompensated under these demanding fixation conditions.

Visual confusion in acquired extraocular muscle palsy

The confusion and dizziness complained of by patients in recently acquired palsy of extraocular muscles is often described in the literature as vertigo or visual vertigo, but it is not true vertigo insomuch as the environment or patient's body does not experience a continuing directional rotation, as occurs in nystagmus from labyrinthine disturbances. There may be a temporary nystagmus if the affected eye attempts to move into the affected field under monocular viewing (*see* below), but in binocular vision the confusion comes about from the changing diplopia. The affected eye's visual image accelerates rapidly in the direction of action of the faulty muscle. The feeling of dizziness, confusion and unsteadiness — even sickness — is due primarily to the increasing diplopia in the field of action of the affected muscle and the associated difficulty in spatial localization in that direction. The environment becomes diplopic and appears to move where the affected muscle cannot cope. Visual confusion is a better description for this experience than vertigo.

Recent paretic ocular deviations are readily determined by the symptoms and by simple objective examination. They suggest vascular, muscular or nervous lesions which require neurological or ophthalmological attention. In long-standing pareses, the acquisition of an abnormal head posture, secondary changes in other muscles and the increasing ability of the patient to avoid version movements into the diplopic field by the simple alternative of making head movements, result in the complaint of confusion being lessened and eventually disappearing.

True nystagmus and vertigo are most likely to arise under monocular viewing conditions when the affected eye attempts to move in the direction of restricted movement. Here, the increasing nervous effort used in an attempt to move the eye results in a jerky nystagmus such as develops normally in extreme eye movements. Under binocular conditions, fixation is usually by the unaffected eye and nystagmus does not develop. The affected eye lags behind and it is then the rapidly changing diplopia which gives the greatest confusion.

Oscillopsia

Oscillopsia is the condition in which the environment appears to move or oscillate[13,14].

Normal causes

Patients sometimes report the intermittent and common clonic blepharospasm of the lower lid as 'vision seeming to twitch'. Pressure on one eye with the fingers causes the environment apparently to move and, in binocular viewing, gives diplopia with one image moving progressively as the pressure is increased. It also occurs from vestibular origin after moving constantly in one direction then stopping. A slow creep occurs in the environment opposite to the previous motion.

Some abnormal causes are given in *Table 12.4*.

TABLE 12.4. Some Causes of Oscillopsia

Clonic blepharospasm (lower lid fibrillar twitch)
Heterophoria
Neurosis
Recent palsy of extraocular muscles
Acquired nystagmus
Multiple sclerosis
Loss of vestibular function

Visual confusion and diplopia

'Sometimes I seem to see double.'
The kind of comment quoted above made calmly by a patient during a history interview suggests that the patient is unlikely to have had persistent binocular diplopia for any length of time. Sudden binocular diplopia causes great confusion and is intolerable to any patient. It also results in alarm, distress and an early call for professional help. The difficulties are emphasized when the angle between the diplopic images is small.

So, patients who have experienced real binocular double vision for more than a brief moment of time will probably describe their experience in more emphatic and definite terms. Nevertheless, a complaint of past double vision can be a very significant indicator for general health, if confirmed, so that however that complaint is phrased, it cannot be disregarded.

If diplopia persists then the patient will find means of avoiding the confusion. Adopting an abnormal head posture may relieve their symptoms either by allowing fusion to take place or by so displacing one of the images that it becomes less obtrusive. More likely, relief will have been obtained by closing off one eye and some form of temporary occlusion will have been carried out varying from the pink plastic eye shades obtainable from the local store to any form of occluding material held in place by various devices. The cosmetic effect is overridden by the urgency of removing the disturbing visual experience of double images. Patients afflicted with very recent binocular diplopia are somewhat unlikely to present themselves in the optometric practice for initial examination, but if they do, then they will often be accompanied by a relative, spouse or friend. In as polite a manner as can be managed it is best to exclude such additional persons from the consulting room.

But, the patient who makes the very casual comment about 'seeing double' may well not have suffered true binocular diplopia at all, or it may have been a normal phenomenon. Some reasons for patients making a comment about double vision are as follows.

Blurred objects are being described as double

Blurred letters or blurred astigmatic fan lines are commonly described as seeming to be double by patients during eye examination. When the distance ametropia is properly corrected then the complaint of double vision disappears, distinguishing true binocular or monocular diplopia from mere blurred imagery. In considering the significance of the complaint of diplopia it is therefore essential first to ensure that simple blurring of objects has been eliminated.

Fatigue effect

Double vision sometimes occurs as a transient phenomenon when a person is tired, as in reading, for example. Accommodation and convergence are both relaxed momentarily resulting in blurring and doubling of near objects for a short time.

Decompensated heterophoria

An existing compensated heterophoria breaks down but is quickly corrected as when some object in the environment acts to disturb fusion and transient diplopia is noticed by the patient.

Physiological diplopia

Rarely will a normal individual notice physiological diplopia although this is sometimes quoted in general texts as one reason for the complaint of double vision. If a normal patient does report diplopia of the physiological variety then he may previously have had orthoptic treatment involving exercises requiring observations of physiological diplopia. The possibility exists that such a patient may have demonstrated the phenomenon to others and the complainant may have thereby developed a neurosis.

Only where it can be shown that refractive correction removes the so-called diplopia (that is, it was confused with blurring) or that it was in some other way spurious or arises from a condition which is under control is the practitioner entitled to conclude that there is no need for further investigation.

Considerations where a patient presents true persistent binocular diplopia

The first action when a patient appears in a state of stress from recently acquired binocular diplopia is for the practitioner to retain composure and to ensure that all the required information is collected from the patient before proceeding to other parts of the examination. The patient will be reassured by a calm attentive and unruffled examiner who shows concern for their worry and distress. It may be obvious within minutes that the patient needs attention outside the immediate sphere of activity of the optometrist but nothing will be gained by omitting to gather the essential information.

The impulse in the newly qualified is to hurry through the initial discussions in order to investigate eye movements by the best available methods; to determine whether a palsy of extraocular muscles has occurred and, in that case, which muscle or muscles

TABLE 12.5. Some Causes of True Binocular Diplopia

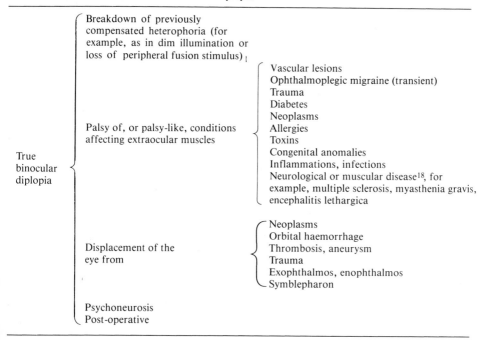

True binocular diplopia

- Breakdown of previously compensated heterophoria (for example, as in dim illumination or loss of peripheral fusion stimulus)
- Palsy of, or palsy-like, conditions affecting extraocular muscles
  - Vascular lesions
  - Ophthalmoplegic migraine (transient)
  - Trauma
  - Diabetes
  - Neoplasms
  - Allergies
  - Toxins
  - Congenital anomalies
  - Inflammations, infections
  - Neurological or muscular disease[18], for example, multiple sclerosis, myasthenia gravis, encephalitis lethargica
- Displacement of the eye from
  - Neoplasms
  - Orbital haemorrhage
  - Thrombosis, aneurysm
  - Trauma
  - Exophthalmos, enophthalmos
  - Symblepharon
- Psychoneurosis
- Post-operative

seem to be affected and then to begin the thought process for writing a letter of referral. There is no surer way to miss some tell-tale symptom or sign than to be carried along on the overriding complaint of diplopia to the exclusion of a proper discussion of the patient's history and other symptoms leading to a normal examination. Only from this data will it be possible to compose a concise and adequate referral report.

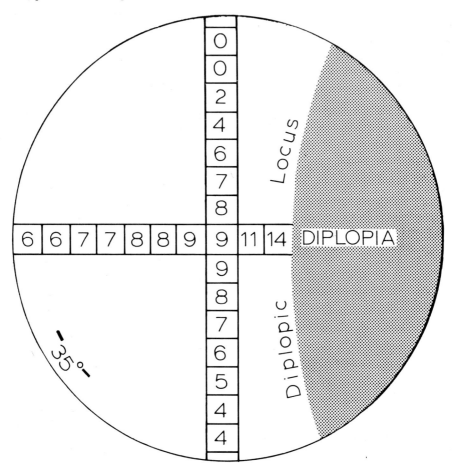

Figure 12.2. Heterophoria and diplopia across the field in long-standing minor paresis of the right external rectus muscle, without symptoms (fixation with unaffected eye). The numbers refer to the esophoric deviation in prism dioptres as measured under dissociation. Binocular diplopia is less pronounced in upward, and to a lesser extent in downward, gaze due to the abducting effects of the oblique muscles. Vertical deviations and cyclorotations are not shown. The condition manifests itself as a moderate esophoria on fixation straight ahead increasing on dextroversion until, at 10–15 degrees, heterotropia intervenes. A right head turn of approximately 10 degrees exists and that normal position is used in the results quoted. Near to the diplopic locus fusion can be maintained only by intense concentration, and widening of the palpebral fissure. When fixing objects to the right, either the head will also be turned to allow fixation to fall within the field of single binocular vision or the right eye is partly or completely closed to help ignore the faulty eye's image (diplopic winking phenomenon). This case example is used to demonstrate that, in minor, long-standing pareses usually from birth, there may be no symptoms described at all in the history symptom interview, yet an extensive diplopic field exists

Sudden, persistent true binocular diplopia points to a muscular, nervous or centrally located lesion. Some indications are given in *Table 12.5*. The minor pareses of extraocular muscles from birth trauma may never be noticed by the patient for they often show up only as a (compensated) heterophoric deviation on the mid-line *(Figure 12.2)*. Later in life some occurrence may demonstrate the double images in a particular direction of gaze and cause the patient concern. The differentiation and detailed investigation of the various forms of binocular diplopia can be found in textbooks devoted to anomalies of binocular vision.

Patients who have recently occluded one eye and who are to continue to do so whilst awaiting further investigations must be warned of the effects of loss of stereopsis and loss of part of their visual field. They must be advised to take care in all activities where these losses introduce hazards such as crossing roads on foot. Driving should be discontinued. In left hand driving rule of the road, occlusion of the right eye eliminates that part of the field in which overtaking vehicles appear. Nevertheless, the main responsibility in such patients is to obtain medical care as soon as this can be arranged.

The presence of true binocular diplopia at the time of examination is easily established if it is not already obvious from the patient's demeanour and/or eye deviation. It is when the patient, who at the time appears normal, reports a history of 'seeing double' that the experience of the practitioner will be taxed. It may have been true and a cause for real concern, yet it may have been spurious. It may have been caused by a quite trivial circumstance such as the prismatic effect of tears or be the first signal of some serious general condition such as multiple sclerosis.

A critical problem-oriented discussion with the patient is vital to determine whether other possible symptoms exist which might give weight to the complaint. As an extreme example it would be no credit to the examiner, nor would the waiting lists of hospitals be helped, if through the action of referral the patient were sent for special investigations when the complaint of seeing double arose from the double images seen normally at the edges of a crescent moon and which simple questioning would have determined. Equally, the patient's interests are best served by certainty in diagnosis.

In general optometric practice the frequency of complaints of double vision in case histories is low and there is a special responsibility to send the patient for general medical examination where any reasonable doubt exists as to the cause of the symptom. Complaints must be treated with suspicion in view of the possibility of demyelinating disease, neoplasms, vascular lesions or diabetes. The main concern should be to attempt to establish whether true binocular diplopia occurred, and where the complaint appears to have substance to initiate procedures for investigation and differential diagnosis.

Monocular diplopia

Except for the confusion with blurred vision, monocular diplopia is uncommon as a presenting symptom in general optometric practice. Where it is complained of its cause is likely to be one of the following conditions (*Table 12.6*).

Irregular refraction

Where there are irregularities in some part of the eye's optical media, notably in the crystalline lens, then secondary images may be complained of. If the secondary retinal

TABLE 12.6. Causes of Monocular Diplopia

Blurred vision only
Spectacle diplopia (for example, bifocal segment edge)

Optical anomalies of the eye	Internal, for example, cataract or pupil abnormality
	External, for example, prismatic effect of tear fluid

Strabismic eyes at certain stages of treatment
Retino-choroidal conditions, for example, retinal separation
Uncommon syndromes of central origin[19]
Psychoneurosis

image or images are far removed from the retinal plane then they will be so blurred as to produce only veiling of the true retinal image, and in such cases will most likely pass unnoticed by the patient or cause reduction in visual acuity, especially in conditions of low luminance.

The most frequent complaints of double or multiple vision arise from crystalline lens changes, particularly senile-type cortical cataract. The spurious images are ill-defined but the effects are especially noticed if the pupil is able to dilate under low brightness conditions so that peripheral areas of the crystalline lens play a greater part in image formation. The irregular refraction can be annoying and hazardous to drivers of motor vehicles for, not only are these ghost images, but the scattering of light over the central region of the retina leads to a general lowering of visual acuity in those conditions.

Posterior subluxation of the crystalline lens

If the crystalline lens has been dislocated from any cause, such that some portion of it still lies within the pupil area and retains its transparency, then monocular diplopia can occur if vision were previously good. The uncorrected aphakic image will be indistinct unless the patient were previously myopic to the order of 10–14 dioptres.

The retinal image formed through the dislocated portion of the lens will also be blurred through the effect of aberrations; the possible tilting of the lens and its greater convexity from the relief of zonular tension. The displaced lens is no longer firmly held within the eye and in the early stages may become further displaced, and show some movement with changes of head position. Secondary changes often follow resulting in the dislocated lens becoming more fixed in position and also opaque so that any complaint of monocular diplopia disappears.

Other optical causes of monocular diplopia

Double pupils or tears in the iris can give rise to diplopic images on the Scheiner disc principle when the retinal images are not exactly focused. Corneal nebulae and other corneal disturbances may cause complaints of diplopia as also can changes in the vitreous humour where areas of altered refractive index occur.

Monocular diplopia in the treatment of strabismus

This form of diplopia develops whilst a long-standing abnormal retinal correspondence is being broken down during orthoptic training. At some stage the patient notices the appearance of a secondary image representing foveal projection in the deviating eye and together with the abnormally corresponding area's image, monocular diplopia then exists in that eye for a time. Diplopia may also persist as a post-operative condition in the correction of strabismus.

References

1 ALEXANDER, K.R. (1975). 'On the nature of accommodative micropsia.' *Am. J. Optom. physiol. Opt.*, **52**, 2, 79–84

2 RICHARDS, W. (1967). 'Apparent modification of receptive fields during accommodation and convergence and a model for size constancy.' *Neuropsychologia*, **5**, 1, 63–72

3 OGLE, K.N. (1962). 'Spatial localisation according to direction.' In *The Eye,* Ed. by DAVSON, H., Vol. 4, p. 227. London: Academic Press

4 PERSONAL OBSERVATIONS

5 FUCHS, E. (1908). *Textbook of Ophthalmology,* 3rd English ed. (Translated by A. DUANE), p. 44. Philadelphia: Lippincott

6 AMSLER, M. (1953). 'Earliest symptoms of disease of the macula.' *Br. J. Ophthal.*, **37**, 521–537

7 CREWS, S.J. (1980). Personal communication

8 HEATON, J.M. (1968). *The Eye. Phenomenology and Psychology of Function and Disorder,* pp. 138–141. London: Tavistock Publications; Philadelphia: Lippincott

9 PERSONAL OBSERVATIONS

10 COGAN, D.G. (1968). 'Down beat nystagmus.' *Archs Ophthal.*, **80**, 757–768

11 NEMA, H.V. (1973). 'Ménière's syndrome.' In *Ophthalmic Syndromes,* pp. 168–169. London: Butterworth

12 HEATON, J.M. (1968). *The Eye. Phenomenology and Psychology of Function and Disorder,* p. 239. London: Tavistock Publications; Philadelphia: Lippincott

13 KROLL, M. (1969). 'Acquired idiopathic nystagmus and oscillopsia.' *Am. J. Ophthal.*, **67**, 139–144

14 BENDER, M.B. (1965). 'Oscillopsia.' *Archs Neurol.*, **13**, 204–213

15 GREEN, H. and SPENCER, J. (1969). *Drugs with Possible Ocular Side Effects.* New York: St. Martin's Press

16 ROY, F.H. (1975). *Ocular Differential Diagnosis,* p. 520. Philadelphia: Lea and Febiger

17 NEMA, H.V. (1973). *Ophthalmic Syndromes.* p. 342. London: Butterworth

18 ROY, F.H. (1975). *Ocular Differential Diagnosis,* p. 526. Philadelphia: Lea and Febiger

19 ROY, F.H. (1975). *Ocular Differential Diagnosis,* p. 527. Philadelphia: Lea and Febiger

Chapter 13

Other problems of patients

During the history and symptom interview, at any time during eye examination or even as the patient is leaving the consulting room office, problems and symptoms are likely to be mentioned, often as a 'throw away' remark which the patient most likely feels is not at all significant. Many *are* found to be without significance but others provide useful and sometimes important indicators to refractive, eye and general conditions.

Thus, the importance of active listening at all times during an examination is once more stressed and it is useful to end this book by re-emphasizing that original comment made in the Preface and in the later Chapters. Each practitioner will no doubt be able to add to the list of problems and symptoms which have been mentioned in the previous Chapters and the final notes below give some concluding information which may stimulate thought in that direction.

Parents' worries about their children's eyes

All of the following complaints from parents relating to their childrens' eyes and vision should be noted and elaborated in discussion[1], followed by the normal refractive and binocular vision examination — frowning, squinting (*see* below), closing one eye in reading, frequent rubbing of eyes, poor performance at school, working at an excessively close distance, intolerance to light, undue difficulty in fast-moving ball games such as football, tennis, cricket, baseball, clumsy behaviour, excess blinking and difficulty in writing or spelling. The last-named dyslexic-type signs are not often eliminated by simply correcting an existing ametropia or binocular vision anomaly. The cause is usually complex but, in the course of investigation and treatment, significant anomalies of binocular vision or refraction should be corrected in accordance with good practice.

Squinting

The common lay use of this word describes the narrowing of the palpebral fissure and furrowing of the forehead as when a person looks towards the bright sky.

'I have brought Johnny in to see you because he squints a lot', is the usual approach. Johnny may be slightly myopic or astigmatic or may 'squint' because his older sister obtained special attention from so doing, and in this case Johnny's refractive state is likely to be within normal limits.

In true intermittent strabismus the parent's comments are usually along the lines of 'eyes turning into the corner', 'appears to have a cast', 'eyes seem to be out of line' or simply 'cross-eyed'.

A simple question to the parent on their use of the word squint resolves the problem.

Holding near work very close

The patient does not usually make this complaint but it arises from the observations and comments of others, particularly parents about their children or teachers about their pupils. Strictly it is more correctly a 'sign' under those circumstances. Reading matter is normally held close by small children for the very obvious reason that their arms are shorter, although in children of school age it can sometimes indicate myopia. Some optical reasons for this problem in older persons includes high hypermetropia, uncorrected myopia, low visual acuity or any condition in which a larger retinal image is beneficial to the patient. High myopes commonly remove their distance glasses or shift them on to the forehead to examine objects or reading matter held around their far point and thereby have a ready means of apparent magnification.

Holding close work further away

This symptom, the classic complaint of the early, uncorrected presbyope, arises not only from the act of holding near work further away but also from a coincidental withdrawal of the head with typical narrowing of the palpebral fissure and furrowing of the forehead. It is one of the few visual symptoms or eye signs recognized by the lay person as indicating the need for reading spectacles and, indirectly, as some crude measure of the age of that individual. The onset of this presbyopic symptom can be psychologically stressful for some patients who realize the age association and causes some, particularly women, to delay examination as long as possible. One of the best ways of helping this type of patient is first to reassure them of the normality of the condition, and secondly to suggest using the near work spectacles in the home for reading, sewing and other similar kinds of activity. The patient readily accepts this advice because of the lack of contact with others in the home. The practitioner knows that this is a first, kindly step only. When the patient experiences the relief of seeing clearly at near distances without strain there is a strong motivating factor in overcoming their reluctance to be seen by others wearing a reading prescription — the ease of seeing overrides the embarrassment.

Occasionally, spectacle wearing patients are found who have come to associate bifocals with the critical age decade of 40–50 years and decline to accept advice on their desirability, much preferring to adapt to distance and near prescriptions made up separately. It is unwise to coerce such patients into a bifocal prescription however much the examiner feels this to be optically needed, unless there is some more profound visual advantage than purely patient convenience. This rarer aversion to bifocals has to be distinguished from the still common belief that 'bifocals are difficult to get used to'. For the majority of patients this is not borne out and reassurance can be given that pronounced and prolonged problems with bifocals is unusual. Whether this is equally true for some recent forms of multifocal lens prescriptions is less certain.

Difficulty in refocusing from near to distance

This problem has been briefly mentioned previously but in young patients, the symptom nearly always indicates a slightly myopic or pseudo-myopic state. The complaint comes typically from a school, college or university student who has to write notes from blackboards or from the distance projections of visual aids. Vision is quite clear for close work but relaxing accommodation for clear distance vision takes much longer than for the average person. The apparent refractive error, when measured, may be a minor degree of myopia as low as 0.25 dioptres determined by the usual methods of examination. Spasm of accommodation in such patients cannot be entirely ruled out although it is often over-stressed in textbooks on refraction. It can be demonstrated under cycloplegia. Without cycloplegics, the pupil size, the muscle balance for distance and near and particularly the presence of hypermetropic-type symptoms of discomfort and possible headache are some indicators to the true refractive state.

Words 'running together' in reading

This is another common symptom of older patients who have developed a large exophoria at near coupled with their diminishing powers of accommodation. It may also occur as a fatigue effect in normal patients during reading and particularly with loss of attention as in dozing. The early presbyope can also present this problem in that the excess accommodative effort used in an attempt to see clearly at near results in some over-convergence for the object of regard. The correct presbyopic addition relieves the problem and for the elderly presbyope, base in prisms prescribed for reading in accordance with good clinical practice, gives relief. Near hyperphoria, sometimes of quite small degree, also leads to this symptom, and may occasionally be induced by the effect of corrected anisometropia in the vertical meridians where there is incorrect centration for near. This is one of the many causes of non-tolerance to an optical prescriptions (Chapter 5).

Fibrillar twitching of the lower lid (myokymia)

This is a very common complaint as a main or secondary symptom for eye examination. Patients complain that their eyelid twitches frequently and not only is this a nuisance and worry to them, but it can be seen when looking into a mirror and friends may remark on the appearance. It is usually associated with personal matters such as overwork, stress, fatigue, insomnia, debility and maybe with refractive errors. The patient should be reassured and ametropia should be corrected in accordance with normal practice.

Dark circles

Patients, usually women, become mildly anxious about the presence of the common dark reddish-brown areas under their eyes. They are noticed by the patient when looking into mirrors and rarely remarked upon directly by other people. If they do so, it is usually to comment that the person 'looks tired'. Because the patient sees them in a reflected image then the illumination is mostly from above, and their appearance is accentuated by shadows. Some are more prone to this kind of appearance than others and, with women, the prominence can be diminished by cosmetics.

A feeling of 'puffy' eyelids which otherwise appear normal on objective examination

This feeling is most pronounced on looking downwards and may be combined with the complaint of dark circles (*see* above). The adnexa may become oedematous in certain well-described conditions such as hyperthyroidism, but the most likely reason for this symptom if there is no obvious sign of lid abnormality and oedema, is over-indulgence, insufficient sleep or stress.

Reference

1 FLOYD WILLIAMS, J. (1976). 'Communicating with parents.' *J. optom. Educ.,* **2,** 1, 1–11

Appendix

Alphabetical reference guide to symptom/problem tables

Certain of the tables are assembled here in alphabetical arrangement with some modifications and additions for quick reference. It is again emphasized that these tables are not exhaustive and intended as a guide only. They refer to possible causes of particular symptoms, many of which might arise in a random catchment urban optometric practice in Great Britain. Space is available for additions and notes and any changes or deletions may be easily carried out.

Index to tables

Blurred Vision

Uncorrected and poorly corrected ametropia and presbyopia
Defects in spectacle lenses
Accommodation/convergence anomalies
Clinical emmetropia with prolonged close work (distance blur)
Migraine
Primary anomalies of the ocular media, for example, nuclear cataract, vitreous haze, irregularity of
  refracting surfaces
Other conditions which decrease the transparency of the ocular media, for example, posterior uveitis
Central retinal oedema, for example, from commotio retinae
Angle closure glaucoma
Nutritional amblyopia
Uncommon syndromes, for example, Posner–Sclossmann

(*See also* Transient blurring below)

Blurred vision — Transient

Mucus passing over cornea
Excess lacrimation (*see* Watering eyes on page 114)
Migraine (*see* Photopsia on page 96)
Vitreous opacities or muscae (*see* Entoptic phenomenon on page 99)

Variable spasm of accommodation
- Convergence excess
- Psychoneuroses
- Irritation of ciliary muscle
- Trauma
- Toxins and drugs
- Irritative IIIrd nerve lesions

Variable insufficiency of accommodation
- Early presbyopia or lens sclerosis
- Pseudo-myopia
- Chronic open angle and chronic angle closure glaucoma
- Drugs and toxins
  - Stimulants
  - Tranquillizers
  - Alcohol
  - Diphtheric
- Trauma
- Diabetes and other general medical conditions

Chronic angle closure glaucoma
Variation in refraction (as in diabetes)
Multiple sclerosis
Functional — IIIrd nerve lesions
Malingering

(*See also* Transient loss of vision on page 142)

Note: Where transient blurring of vision is given in the history and not evident at the time of examination then the blurring complained of may have been a real loss of vision, usually central.

Diplopia — Binocular

True binocular diplopia
- Breakdown of previously compensated heterophoria (for example, as in dim illumination or loss of peripheral fusion stimulus)
- Palsy of, or palsy-like, conditions affecting extraocular muscles
  - Vascular lesions
  - Ophthalmoplegic migraine (transient)
  - Trauma
  - Diabetes
  - Neoplasms
  - Allergies
  - Toxins
  - Congenital anomalies
  - Inflammations, infections
  - Neurological, or muscular disease, for example, multiple sclerosis, myasthenia gravis, encephalitis lethargica
- Displacement of the eye from
  - Neoplasms
  - Orbital haemorrhage
  - Thrombosis, aneurysm
  - Trauma
  - Exophthalmos, enophthalmos
  - Symblepharon
- Psychoneurosis
- Post-operative

Diplopia — Monocular

Blurred vision only
Spectacle diplopia (for example, bifocal segment edge)

Optical anomalies of the eye
- Internal, for example, cataract or pupil abnormality
- External, for example, prismatic effect of tear fluid

Strabismic eyes at certain stages of treatment
Retino-choroidal conditions, for example, retinal separation
Uncommon syndromes of central origin
Psychoneurosis

Discomfort — In or Around the Eyes

WHITE EYE(S)

With no significant hyperaemia in uncomplicated cases

Minor psychological stresses
Use of eyes in prolonged exacting visual tasks
Ametropia, presbyopia
Binocular vision anomalies
Sinus/nasal problems
Contact lenses
Glaucoma — open angle (often symptomless)
Early retrobulbar neuritis
Glaucoma — chronic angle closure
Hysteria
Malingering

With superficial hyperaemia in uncomplicated cases

Irritants
Lack of sleep
Climate: cold, wind, sun
Contact lenses
Ametropia, presbyopia
Binocular vision anomalies
Eyelash in punctum or in conjunctival sac
Other minor foreign bodies
Allergies including conjunctival mucus (as in hay fever)
Pinguecula
Styes
Reduction in tear flow or lack of fluid reaching conjunctival sac
Minor trauma
Sinus/nasal infections
Concretions
Trichiasis
Glaucoma — chronic angle closure
Nutritional deficiencies
Malingering (self-administered drugs/chemicals)

Subconjunctival haemorrhage (commonly without discomfort)

'Dry' eye(s)

Age changes
Allergies
Toxins, drugs
Anomalies of lacrimal/conjunctival glands
Some forms of conjunctivitis
Nutritional deficiencies
Infrequent blinking
Some systemic diseases
Rare syndromes

RED EYE(S)

With marked hyperaemia superficial and/or deep

Loose or embedded foreign body
Corneal abrasions
Conjunctivitis: chronic/acute in its many forms
Allergies
Excess exposure to ultraviolet radiation
Sinus/nasal infections
Other corneal afflictions: ulceration, keratitis
Trauma
Blepharitis: chronic/acute in its many forms
Acute iridocyclitis
Infections of lacrimal apparatus
Acute glaucoma
Scleritis and episcleritis
Tumours
Malingering

Note: Discomfort may, or may not, be described in terms of 'pain' (*see* page 110).

Dizziness (Mild Vertigo-type Sensations usually Without Nystagmus and With No Sense of Continuing Directional Rotation)

Effects of heights
Heterophoria and pareses of extraocular muscles
Recently corrected refractive errors causing spatial distortion
Some forms of bifocal and multifocal correction in susceptible patients
Circulatory problems as in fainting
Accommodation spasms
Metamorphopsia, refractive or retinal
Adverse effect of drugs

Dry Eye

Age changes
Allergies
Toxins, drugs
Some forms of conjunctivitis
Anomalies of lacrimal/conjunctival glands
Nutritional deficiencies
Infrequent blinking from any cause
Some systemic diseases
Sjögren's syndrome

Floaters

Non-pathological embryonic remnants
Myopia
Separation or adhesion of vitreous humour (shrinkage retraction)
Fluidity of vitreous humour
Vitreous haemorrhage
Retinal detachment
Uveitis
Foreign bodies (mostly in posterior vitreous humour except under special viewing conditions)

Note: Asteroid bodies (asteroid hyalitis) and synchisis scintillans rarely give rise to the symptom of floaters. Where the complaint of floaters appears to indicate a sudden origin or sudden rapid increase then some condition such as retinal separation must be suspected.

Halos

Physiological from radial structure of crystalline lens
Environmental (vision through condensation on glass, etc.)
Pathological from corneal oedema as from chronic angle closure glaucoma

Headache

Relatively common in general optometric practice	Relatively uncommon or rare in general optometric practice
Stress, muscular tension, anxiety, depression, overwork, insomnia	Chronic angle closure glaucoma
	Retrobulbar neuritis
Over-indulgence, addiction (for example alcohol)	Raised intracranial pressure, brain abscess, tumour
Fatigue, constipation	
Uncorrected or poorly corrected refractive errors	Ocular inflammations
Accommodation anomalies, heterophoria and other binocular vision anomalies	Fever, inflammation of cranial arteries
	Subarachnoid bleeding
Undue physical activity	Intracranial aneurysms
Migraine and its variants	Otitis
Adverse effects of drugs, toxins, exogenous, endogenous	Severe trauma
	Encephalitis
Vascular hypertension	Deficiency diseases
Minor trauma	
Foci of infection, oral, nasal sinuses	

Loss of Vision — Bilateral, Central

Migraine (paracentral)
Toxins and drugs (for example, methanol, chronic ethyl alcoholism, lead, etc.)
Macular degeneration
'Eclipse' blindness
Bilateral central retinal oedema
Retrobulbar neuritis, bilateral
Trauma
Nutritional amblyopia
Cortical lesions

Loss of Vision — Unilateral, Central

Vitreous opacity
Optic neuritis, acute axial neuritis, retrobulbar neuritis
Macular degeneration or haemorrhage
Central choroiditis
Commotio retinae and other trauma

Loss of Vision — Unilateral, Sudden, Total

Haemorrhage into the vitreous humour
Occlusion of central retinal artery
Retinal detachment (occurring overnight, it may appear to have been sudden)
Trauma
Acute glaucoma
Functional

(*See also* 'Central' visual loss above)

Loss of Vision — Transient

Mucus passing over the cornea (as in hay fever)
Excess lacrimation
Gravitational effects (as in stooping and rising rapidly)
Migraine
Vitreous opacities
Retinal vascular disease, including embolic and spastic episodes
Chronic angle closure glaucoma
Interference of blood supply to optic nerve (for example, raised I.O.P.)
Hypotension (fundal, as in papilloedema)
Vascular insufficiency (for example, carotid artery syndrome)
Optic neuritis, retrobulbar neuritis (as in multiple sclerosis)
Trauma, such as a blow on the eye
General systemic conditions (for example, hypertension)
Functional
Malingering

(*See also* Blurring)

Note: Where transient loss of vision is given in the history, and not evident at the time of examination, then the 'loss' may have been incomplete or there may have been visual blur only.

Metamorphopsia — Regular and irregular

Metamorphopsia, general	Physiological, for example, strong accommodation/convergence Refractive Retinal Neurological Drugs, toxins
Irregular metamorphopsia	Vision through prisms Media irregularities Central retinal oedema Macular degeneration Central lesions
Macropsia	Vision through hazy atmosphere Recently corrected presbyopia, hypermetropia Base-in prisms and other optical devices Spasm of accommodation
Micropsia	Vision in very clear atmospheres Base-out prisms and other optical devices Recently corrected myopia Neurosis, psychosis Intoxication Palsy of accommodation Occipital and parietal lobe lesions
Pelopsia	Recent optical corrections (for example, presbyopic additions) Vision in very clear atmospheres Neurosis, psychosis
Teleopsia	Vision in hazy atmospheres In drowsiness (transient) Occipital and parietal lobe lesions Intoxication (varians) Neurosis, psychosis (usually transient)

Night Vision — Defective

	Possible cause	*State of adaptometric terminal threshold, if measured*
Poor vision at low luminance levels	Uncorrected or poorly corrected refractive errors, especially myopia	Normal or near normal
	Age effect of small pupils	Normal or near normal
	Peripheral lens changes as in early senile-type cortical cataract	Probably within normal limits for the patient's age unless the condition is advanced
	Peripheral corneal irregularities	Probably within normal limits
	Some forms of glaucoma	Probably abnormal
	Retinitis pigmentosa and its variations	Highly abnormal as an early characteristic in both recessive and dominant inheritance
	Psychological problems including hysteria	Probably normal but may show fluctuations
	Congenital nyctalopia	No scotopic function
	Metabolic disorders including avitaminosis A Liver disease	Elevation of terminal threshold at some stage dependent on the individual
	Rare syndromes (for example, Uyemura's)	

Non-tolerance to Prescriptions — Some Possible Causes

Dispensing errors, for example, incorrect effective power, centration or positioning of bifocal segment edge
Inappropriate use of prescription
Patient adaptation phenomenon, for example, unaccustomed cylinders or prisms, recently corrected myopia, presbyopia
Dispensing problems, for example, reflections from lens surfaces, lens edge thickness, visibility of bifocal segment, overall weight, change of previously worn lens form, colour, type of frame, deletion of previously worn, and apparent, tint
Errors in final prescription, for example, uncorrected residual errors, imbalance in prescription giving marginal monocular blur, unintended prismatic effects
Undetected or subsequently developed eye or eye-related disease
Faulty management of patient and/or initial examination
Patient dissatisfaction with practitioner, initial examination, attention from auxiliary personnel, inability to pay

Oscillopsia

Clonic blepharospasm (lower lid fibrillar twitch)
Heterophoria
Neurosis
Recent palsy of extraocular muscles
Acquired nystagmus
Multiple sclerosis
Loss of vestibular function

Peripheral Visual Loss — Total/partial

Migraine (transient and partial)
Glaucoma, especially open angle, later stages
Toxic amblyopia (for example, quinine, chloroquine, arsenic, carbon monoxide)
Retinitis pigmentosa and its variants
Peripheral choroiditis
Chiasmal lesions such as bitemporal hemianopia and its variants
Retrochiasmal lesions, such as homonymous hemianopia and its variants
Trauma (for example, to occipital lobe as in double homonymous hemianopia with macular sparing)
Some forms of optic atrophy (for example, tabetic)
Bilateral occlusion of the central retinal arteries with cilio-retinal central retention (unusual)
Hysteria

Peripheral Visual Loss — Apparent (Usually Partial)

Spectacle frames, lens faults
Change in postural habits: headwear, hairstyle
High prescriptions, as in aphakia
Environmental factors, especially in performing special visual tasks
Acquired ptosis
Malingering
Miosis

Photophobia

	Hay fever
	Mydriasis from drugs and other causes
	Functional
	Corneal irritation (for example, foreign body in conjunctival sac)
Generally mild	Contact lens wear
	Myopia
	Migraine
	Trigeminal irritability
	Post-operative aphakia
	Retrobulbar neuritis
	Anterior segment lesions (for example, keratoconjunctivitis, iridocyclitis, corneal ulceration, iritis)
	Toxins and adverse effects of drugs
	Buphthalmos
Generally severe	Febrile conditions
	Partial or total aniridia
	Albinism
	Achromatopsia
	Obsessional psychogenic

Photopsia

Entoptic effects (for example, phosphenes, gravitational or 'blow' phenomenon)
Migraine
Adverse effects of drugs
Retinal, choroidal and optic nerve conditions
Occipital cranial lesions, other than migraine
Epilepsy

Vertigo — True, with Jerky Nystagmus and Subjective Directional Sense of Rotation

Physiological, from artificial labyrinthine stimulation
Ménière's syndrome
Pathological nystagmus of peripheral or central origin, for example:
    Acute labyrinthitis
    Lesions of vestibular pathways
    Raised intracranial pressure
    Multiple sclerosis
    Lesions of brain stem or cerebellum
    Vascular lesions
Adverse effect of drugs or toxins, for example, alcohol

Visual Unease

Mucus passing over the cornea
Need for change in optical prescription, often unilateral
Uncorrected ametropia, usually minor and unilateral
Minor stresses in binocular fusion or accommodation
Effect of drugs and toxins
Loss of contrast sensitivity (demyelinating disease, glaucoma, diabetes)
Epilepsy
Neurological lesions
Psychological disorders

Watering Eyes

Cold, wind, sun (especially older patients)
Emotion, pain
Foreign body: loose, embedded
Corneal abrasion
Irritants (especially in industry) and allergies
Misplacement of punctum (especially older patients)
Ametropia, presbyopia, binocular vision anomalies
Conjunctivitis of some form
Other corneal afflictions, for example, ulceration
Lacrimal gland anomalies
Obstruction to tear drainage
Rare syndromes

Additional reading suggestions

These additional texts may be useful for follow-up study

BOYNTON, R.M. (1979). *Human Colour Vision.* New York: Holt, Rinehart and Winston
HABER, R.N. and HERSHENSON, M. (1974). *The Psychology of Visual Perception,* (int. ed.). London: Holt, Rinehart and Winston
MAUSOLF, F.A. (Ed.) (1980). *The Eye and Systemic Disease,* 2nd ed. St. Louis: Mosby
MICHAELS, D.D. (1980). *Visual Optics and Refraction — A Clinical Approach.* St. Louis: Mosby
O'CONNOR DAVIES, P.H. (1981). *The Actions and Uses of Ophthalmic Drugs,* 2nd. ed. London: Butterworth
PAU, H. (1978). *Differential Diagnosis of Eye Disease,* translated by CIBIS, G. Philadelphia: Saunders
RECORDS, R.E. (Ed.) (1979). *Physiology of the Eye and Visual System.* Hagerstown, MD: Harper and Row
WALSH, T.J. (1978). *Neuro-ophthalmology: Clinical Signs and Symptoms.* Philadelphia: Lea and Febiger

Index